Contemporary Management of Lower Extremity Aneurysmal Disease

Sachinder Singh Hans

Contemporary Management of Lower Extremity Aneurysmal Disease

Springer

Sachinder Singh Hans
Vascular and Endovascular Services
Henry Ford Macomb Hospital
Clinton Township, MI, USA

ISBN 978-3-032-00158-0 ISBN 978-3-032-00159-7 (eBook)
https://doi.org/10.1007/978-3-032-00159-7

This Springer imprint is published by the registered company Springer Nature Switzerland AG
The registered company address is: Gewerbestrasse 11, 6330 Cham, Switzerland

Foreword

Welcome to the *Contemporary Management of Lower Extremity Aneurysmal Diseases*. I would like to congratulate Dr. Sachinder Hans for organizing a phenomenal team of editors and contributors for this text. The guidance provided by them is truly from experts in the field who have a wealth of knowledge and clinical experience.

There are a growing number of texts related to vascular disease and its medical and surgical management. Most of these books are referenced sporadically in day-to-day practice, and they often remain on the shelf. This is a text, however, that is likely to remain open on your desk. The 22 chapters are organized to provide epidemiologic background, patient management and technical information enhanced by the inclusion of spectacular colored images. A very helpful aspect of the chapters is the inclusion of case examples, which contextualizes the academic information into real-world practice.

In a broader view, the textbook focuses on the management of different types of lower extremity aneurysms. It is not merely a collection of facts and procedures, but it is an essential resource that equips clinicians with the tools they need to think critically and act decisively in the management of lower extremity aneurysmal disease. Throughout the chapters, the authors provide valuable insights into the nuances of evaluating aneurysms of the iliac, femoral, popliteal, and distal arteries, with an emphasis on both clinical and radiological assessment. The book also addresses critical complications associated with aneurysmal disease, such as the risk of thrombosis, embolism, and rupture. It is rare to have lower extremity aneurysmal disease as the focus of an entire book, and these topics are frequently not covered in this depth and can be "lost" in the midst of other important topics. Its focus is one of the keystones to the usefulness of this text.

As you navigate through its pages, I suspect that you will find this textbook an indispensable resource in treating patients with lower extremity aneurysmal disease. It will be useful for all stages of careers—from trainees to established surgeons and interventionalists. Again, congratulations to Dr. Hans and colleagues.

Matthew J. Eagleton

Preface

Lower extremity aneurysmal disease has attracted considerably less attention as compared to lower extremity occlusive disease despite the potential for serious complications if not properly diagnosed and managed. This was the impetus to write a short book on this important topic. The first two chapters describe the history of aneurysmal disease and the surgical anatomy followed by chapters on noninvasive, duplex imaging, CTA, MRA, and catheter-based arteriography. Extravascular and open surgical repair of femoral, femoral anastomotic, popliteal artery, infrapopliteal aneurysms, mycotic femoral artery aneurysms, and popliteal venous aneurysms are covered in detail. Femoral and popliteal arterial-venous fistulas, with and without aneurysmal disease, are described. Invited commentaries from distinguished vascular surgeons, radiologists, and interventional radiologists complement the text in most chapters. The last chapter of multiple choice questions highlight some of the important information in each chapter.

The author is grateful to all the contributors of invited commentary for their valuable time, sharing their experience, and providing some extremely useful information to the readers. My sincere thanks to Kris Spring (Managing Editor—Springer) for his unflinching support and seeing the value of this book. Melanie Bednarski, MLIS, Henry Ford Macomb Hospital Librarian, has been a major asset in the completion of the final product, and I am extremely grateful to her for her splendid performance. I am extremely appreciative of Robert Garza former editor of Wayne State University Bulletin for providing editorial assistance. Dr. Gulbash Chandok, OBE and a well-respected General Practitioner from Southall, UK, provided specimen pictures of the popliteal artery aneurysm from Hunterian museum and for that I am highly appreciative. Finally, my sincere thanks to Shanmugapriya Kaliyamoorthy (Production Editor—Springer) for her prompt response to our emails and keeping the process on course.

I sincerely hope that the readers will find this book useful in their clinical practice so that our patients with lower extremity aneurysmal disease are optimally managed.

Clinton Township, MI, USA — Sachinder Singh Hans

Contents

The original version of the book has been revised. A correction to this book can be found at https://doi.org/10.1007/978-3-032-00159-7_23

Commentary Authors

Anahita Dua, MD, MS, MBA Division of Vascular and Endovascular Surgery, Massachusetts General Hospital/Harvard Medical School, Boston, MA, USA

Milan V. Pantelic, MD, MSE, FACR Body MRI, Henry Ford Hospital/Health Network, Henry Ford West Bloomfield Hospital, West Bloomfield, MI, USA

Radiology, Wayne State School of Medicine, Detroit, MI, USA

Shehbaz Shaikh, MD Vascular and Interventional Radiology, Henry Ford Health System, Detroit, MI, USA

Animesh Rathore, MD, RPVI Division of Vascular Surgery, Department of Surgery, Macon and Joan Brock Virginia Health Sciences Center at Old Dominion University, Norfolk, VA, USA

NavYash Gupta, MD, FACS Division of Vascular Surgery, Cedars-Sinai Medical Center, Los Angeles, CA, USA

Dipankar Mukherjee, MD, FACS, DFSVS Vascular Surgery, Inova Fairfax Hospital, Falls Church, VA, USA

Daniel J. Reddy, MD, FACS Wayne State University School of Medicine, Detroit, MI, USA

Raghu Motaganahalli, MD, RPVI, FRCS, FACS, DFSVS Vascular Surgery, Indiana University School of Medicine, Indianapolis, IN, USA

Mitchell Weaver, MD, FACS Henry Ford Hospital, Detroit, MI, USA

Wayne State University School of Medicine, Detroit, MI, USA

Krish Soundarajan, MD, MBA Vascular Surgery, Queens Hospital Center, Queens, NY, USA

QA and Performance Improvement at Mount Sinai Health Center, New York, NY, USA

Paul Bove, MD, FACS Surgery, Oakland University William Beaumont School of Medicine, Royal Oak, MI, USA

Sashi Inkollu, MD Limb Preservation Program, University of Southern Florida, Tampa, FL, USA

Peter Henke, MD Vascular Surgery, University of Michigan, Ann Arbor, MI, USA

Tamer N. Boules, MD Vascular Surgery, Henry Ford Medical Group, Henry Ford West Bloomfield Hospital, West Bloomfield, MI, USA

Ravi Rajani, MD, FACS Grady Memorial Hospital, Emory University School of Medicine, Atlanta, GA, USA

Animesh Rathore, MD Division of Vascular Surgery, Department of Surgery, Macon and Joan Brock Virginia Health Sciences Center at Old Dominion University, Norfolk, VA, USA

History of Lower Extremity Aneurysmal Disease

1

In the *Ebers Papyrus* which is among the earliest medical notations and probably compiled around 2000 BC, the identification of arterial aneurysms—most likely peripheral aneurysms—was described [1–3]. The recommended treatment therein was to treat it with a knife and cauterize it with fire so that it did not bleed "too much." Antyllus, a second-century prominent physician and surgeon, described two forms of these lesions: those originating from a local dilatation in an artery, which were cylindrical, and those resulting from trauma, which were rounded. He described the proximal and distal ligation of the arteries that entered and left the aneurysm, cutting into the aneurysm sac, evacuating its contents, and packing the cavity. There were few advances made in the treatment of aneurysm in the following millenniums until Ambroise Paré (1510–1590) advocated the application of a proximal ligature to an aneurysm [1, 3]. He did not advocate opening the sac of the aneurysm for fear of fatal hemorrhage. The first three recorded successful cases involving this procedure were described by Guanttani in 1772 [1, 3]. Subsequently, Theodore Maunoir from Switzerland (1806–1869) described a flexion technique of the hip and knee joint, together and separately, to induce thrombosis; Sir Walter Reid RN in 1875 described the Esmarch bandage technique with a success rate of slightly over 50%. Indirect pressure—either digital, applied by trained assistants, the use of weights up to 12 lbs. in the thigh, or instrumental pressure with a device with one or more screws tightened on the femoral artery in the groin or the thigh—was employed. This manual form of compression was successful in 47% of cases. The overall death and amputation rate was 7.5%.

On June 22, 1785, Pierre-Joseph Desault ligated popliteal artery as it entered a popliteal aneurysm at Hotel-Dieu in Paris. With John Hunter, surgery began to emerge as a scientific discipline based on the fundamentals of anatomy, physiology, and pathology. He opened the first school of anatomy in Covent Garden in London. In addition to his clinical studies, he studied compression therapy to induce thrombosis in the popliteal aneurysm either indirectly on the aneurysm or on the SFA. The growth of collateral circulation of occluded main arteries gave an impetus for treating aneurysms. On December 12, 1785, Hunter performed SFA ligation of the

S. S. Hans, *Contemporary Management of Lower Extremity Aneurysmal Disease*,
https://doi.org/10.1007/978-3-032-00159-7_1

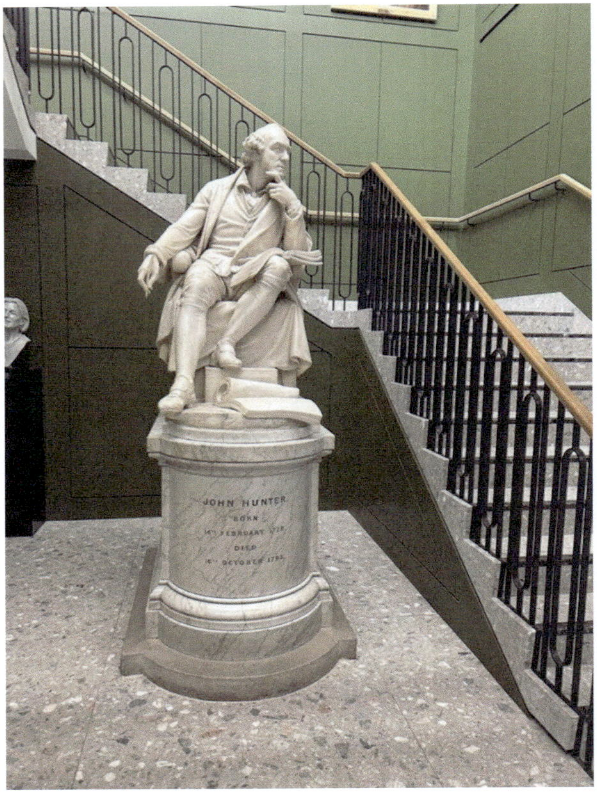

Fig. 1.1 Statue of John Hunter at the Hunterian Museum, London, UK

proximal thigh in the adductor canal (now also known as Hunter's canal) to treat popliteal aneurysm [1, 3] (Fig. 1.1).

He ligated the SFA with four ligatures but did not evacuate the contents of the aneurysm and left the wound open to heal by secondary intention. The patient did well but died 15 months later due to unrelated causes. Hunter performed the autopsy and confirmed that there was no suppuration at the ligature site. The specimen of the popliteal artery aneurysm is preserved in the Hunterian Museum, London (Fig. 1.2a, b).

Hunter treated four more patients with popliteal artery aneurysms in the same fashion with only one failure. Autopsy on one of his patients many years after treatment of popliteal aneurysm repair showed that the entire SFA and popliteal artery were converted into a solid cord. Based on his experiments on canine femoral artery, Hunter ligated a relatively healthy SFA proximal to the aneurysm and concluded that pathology of aneurysmal disease was in the vessel wall and was local in nature. He was cognizant of the importance of collaterals and did not want to disturb the collateral flow concept, which was relatively new during that time [1, 3].

Astley Cooper, a medical student, had studied the effects of brachial and femoral artery ligation in dogs. In 1808, he doubly ligated and divided the common carotid

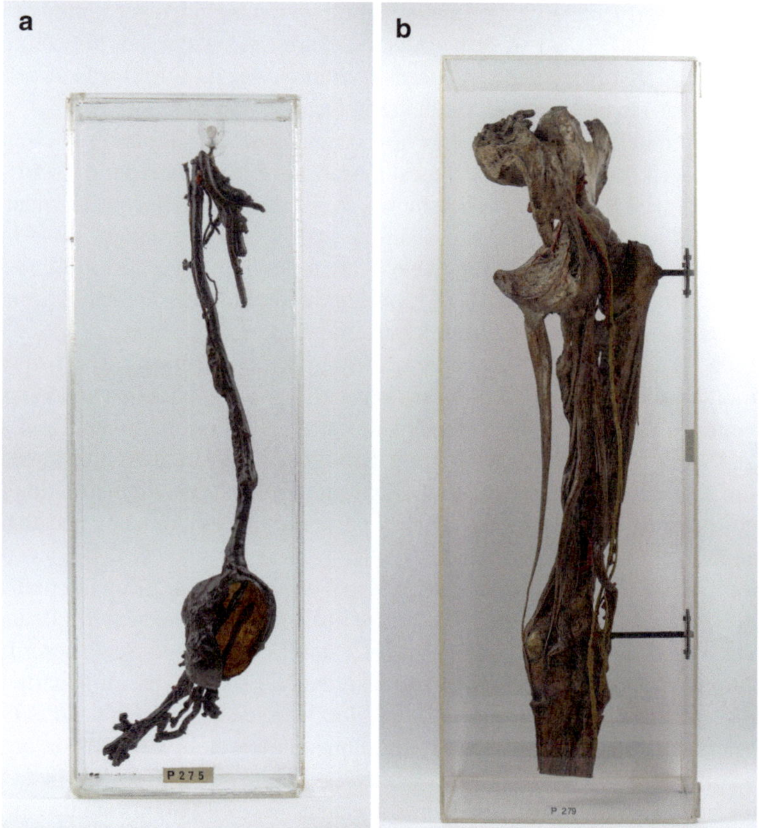

Fig. 1.2 (**a**) Specimen of the ligated popliteal aneurysm. (**b**) Specimen of the leg which had the ligated popliteal aneurysm procedure with kind permission from the Royal College of Surgeons of England

artery proximal to the walnut-sized left carotid aneurysm. (The patient survived until 1821 but eventually died of left-sided cerebral hemorrhage.) Cooper also performed ligation of an external iliac artery for a large femoral aneurysm, and the patient lived until 1826. He also performed ligation of distal abdominal aorta for a very large external iliac aneurysm with the use of a buried catgut suture for ligation in 1817, but the patient died 40 h later. In Australia, Andrew Gibson ligated the femoral artery under preoperative doses of alcohol and opium, 1 inch above the aneurysm just below the inguinal ligament without any distal ischemia on October 25, 1827; however, a secondary hemorrhage ensued over the next few weeks [1, 3]. Gibson performed proximal ligation of the external iliac artery above the groin and femoral artery below the aneurysm [4]. The circulation of the limb was intact until the patient's death in 1828 after about 6 months post operation.

In 1904, Alexis Carrel, a French surgeon, moved to Montreal. He presented a paper on vascular anastomosis. Carrèl and Charles Claude Guthrie of the University of Chicago performed their experimental work, which included perfection of vascular anastomosis and the use of vein grafts in the arterial system. For his accomplishments in vascular surgery and renal transplantation, Alexis Carrel was awarded the Nobel Prize for Physiology and Medicine in October 1912 [1, 3].

The very first clinical anastomosis of a venous graft into the arterial circulatory system was performed by José Goyanes of Madrid in 1906 for a patient with syphilitic popliteal aneurysm. The aneurysm was excised, and an adjacent segment of the popliteal vein was used as an interposition graft [1, 3]. Bernheim, in 1915, performed an interposition saphenous vein graft following the excision of syphilitic popliteal aneurysm. Kunlin, in 1949, reported the first use of saphenous vein grafts as a bypass conduit for lower extremity arterial disease.

In 1896, Wilhelm Conrad Roentgen reported his discovery of x-rays in *Nature*, and 3 months later, the first arteriogram was performed by Haschek and Lindenthal by injecting a radiopaque mixture into the arteries of an amputated arm to test Roentgen's discovery. In 1924, Barney Brooks used sodium iodide injection to study the arterial anatomy of the lower extremities. In 1929, Reynaldo dos Santos reported the arteriography of the abdominal aorta and its branches and the lower extremities.

Thrombosis as the most significant problem with bypass grafting led to the laboratory discovery of heparin in 1916 by a medical student named Jay McLean, but it was too toxic for clinical use at the time [1]. In 1933, Best and Scott described the purification of heparin. In 1940, Murray described the clinical use of heparin for the prevention of thrombosis during repair of blood vessels [1]. In 1946, John Cid dos Santos performed the first successful thromboendarterectomy. Exclusion or partial excision of popliteal aneurysms with saphenous vein bypass grafts had been a standard operation for almost 60 years until the first use of a Palmaz stent with PTFE (polytetrafluoroethylene) graft to treat symptomatic popliteal artery aneurysm exclusion (PA) in 1994 as an endovascular technique.

Recently, the results from a multinational multicenter registry were reported comparing endovascular repair (ER) with open surgical repair (OSR). The perioperative complication rate was low after ER as compared to OSR. The most frequent postoperative complication was impaired wound healing and major bleeding after OSR. The inhospital length of stay was longer for the OSR group [5]. The overall patency rate for the OSR and ER groups after 12 was 83.2% and 44% ($p < 0.005$) respectively and at 24 months 74.2% and 29.1% ($p < 0.005$) respectively. The outcomes with a prosthetic graft versus autologous vein were significantly poorer in the OSR group (primary patency 71.4% vs. 88% at 12 months) [5].

References

1. Friedman SG. A history of vascular surgery. Oxford: Wiley; 2008.
2. Thompson JE. Early history of aortic surgery. J Vasc Surg. 1998;28(4):746–52. https://doi.org/10.1016/s0741-5214(98)70107-7.
3. Galland RB. History of the management of popliteal artery aneurysms. Eur J Vasc Endovasc Surg. 2008;35(4):466–72. https://doi.org/10.1016/j.ejvs.2007.11.011.

4. Mellick SA. The birth of vascular surgery in Australia. J Vasc Surg. 2012;55(4):1213–6. https://doi.org/10.1016/j.jvs.2011.12.011.
5. Jung G, Leinweber ME, Karl T, Geisbüsch P, Balzer K, Schmandra T, Dietrich T, Derwich W, Gray D, Schmitz-Rixen T. Real-world data of popliteal artery aneurysm treatment: analysis of the POPART registry. J Vasc Surg. 2022;75(5):1707–1717.e1702. https://doi.org/10.1016/j.jvs.2021.12.079.

Surgical Anatomy of the Lower Extremity Vascular System

2

The Lower Extremity Vascular System is Comprised of Arteries, Veins, and Lymphatics

Arteries The Arteries of the Lower Extremity anatomically start from the origin of the common iliac artery (CIA) anterior and to the left of the fourth lumbar vertebral body. The CIA bifurcates into the external iliac artery (EIA) and internal iliac artery (IIA). The EIA exits the pelvis under the inguinal ligament to become the common femoral artery (CFA). The common femoral artery courses lateral to the femoral vein, and the femoral nerve courses lateral to the common femoral artery. The mean diameter of the femoral artery is 9.8 mm in men and 8.2 mm in women [1]. The common femoral artery length is often variable. Common femoral artery, vein, and femoral canal are embedded within the femoral sheath (Fig. 2.1).

The femoral canal is a potential space and contains lymph nodes with associated lymphatic vessels. The CFA is the main arterial supply of the lower extremity and is approximately 4 cm in length. It gives off a large branch in the proximal thigh—the profunda femoris or deep femoral artery—and continues as the superficial femoral artery passing into the posterior compartment of the thigh through an opening in the adductor magnus to become the popliteal artery. In the proximal thigh, below the groin, the femoral artery is in the femoral triangle and below the femoral triangle in the adductor (subsartorial or Hunter) canal.

Variations The length of the CFA is often variable with bifurcation into the profunda femoris (deep femoral artery) and the SFA. Occasionally, the common femoral artery divides below the origin of the deep femoral artery into two trunks, which reunite near the opening in the adductor magnus muscle. Occasionally, it is absent, being replaced by inferior gluteal artery, which accompanies the sciatic nerve to the popliteal fossa. This is due to the persistence of the upper part of the original axis artery, with the external iliac artery being rudimentary and ending as the deep femoral artery (persistent sciatic artery). In the complete form of this anomaly, the

S. S. Hans, *Contemporary Management of Lower Extremity Aneurysmal Disease*,
https://doi.org/10.1007/978-3-032-00159-7_2

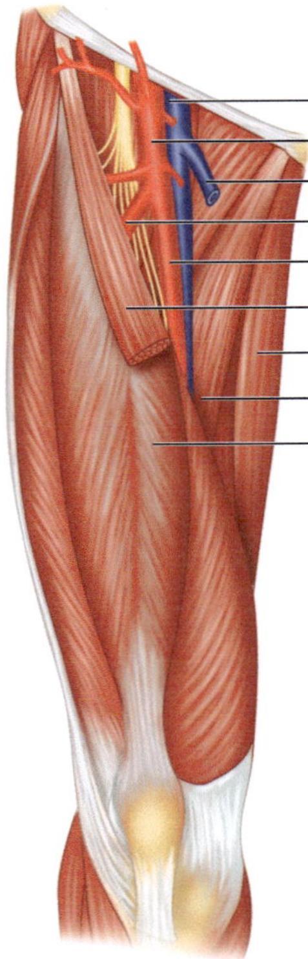

Fig. 2.1 Anatomy of the femoral vessels in the upper thigh

internal iliac artery exits the pelvis through the sciatic foramen, descends in the posterior thigh (adjacent to the sciatic nerve), and continues as the popliteal artery. The deep femoral artery is usually preserved, and the SFA is hypoplastic in more than 60% of the cases, often dividing into terminal branches in the distal thigh. Persistent sciatic arteries are tortuous, often show diffuse enlargement, and are associated with aneurysm formation in more than 25% of the reported cases [1].

Branches

1. Superficial epigastric artery
2. Superficial circumflex iliac artery
3. Superficial external pudendal artery
4. Deep external pudendal artery
5. Muscular branches

Deep Femoral Artery (Profunda Femoris Artery)

This is a large branch arising from the posterior lateral aspect of the CFA 3.5 cm below the inguinal ligament. At first, lateral to the CFA/SFA, the profunda femoris runs behind the SFA with the femoral vein on its medial side and descends between the adductor longus and adductor magnus with its terminal portion, which is sometimes named as a fourth perforating artery [1].

Variations Deep femoral artery (profunda femoris) sometimes arises from the medial side of the CFA and very rarely posteriorly from the CFA. The distance from the inguinal ligament to the origin of the vessel is often variable but is usually 2.5–5 cm below the inguinal ligament. The deep femoral artery establishes several important collateral anastomoses with the internal and external iliac arteries above and the popliteal artery below in the presence of SFA occlusive disease.

Branches
1. Lateral circumflex femoral artery
2. Medial circumflex femoral artery
3. Perforating arteries

Superficial femoral artery, besides giving muscular branches, gives off descending genicular artery just before it passes through the adductor magnus tendon.

The Popliteal Artery

The popliteal artery is the continuation of the superficial femoral artery and traverses the popliteal fossa. It begins at the opening in the adductor magnus (hiatus magnus) at the junction of the middle and distal thirds of the thigh and courses inferiorly and laterally to the intercondylar fossa of the femur. At the lower border of the popliteus muscle anterior tibial artery (ATA) arises at an angle at which; and the popliteal artery continues as the tibial-peroneal trunk and dividing into the posterior tibial (PT) and peroneal artery [1].

Variations Occasionally, the popliteal artery divides into terminal branches above the level of the popliteus, and the anterior tibial artery descends anterior to it. The popliteal artery may divide into anterior tibial (AT) and peroneal arteries, with posterior tibial artery (PTA) being rudimentary or absent. Occasionally, the popliteal artery divides into three branches, i.e., the anterior tibial, the PT, and the peroneal arteries—the so-called trifurcation [1] (Fig. 2.2).

Branches
1. Muscular and cutaneous branches
2. Sural arteries
3. Superior genicular arteries
4. Middle genicular artery
5. Inferior genicular arteries

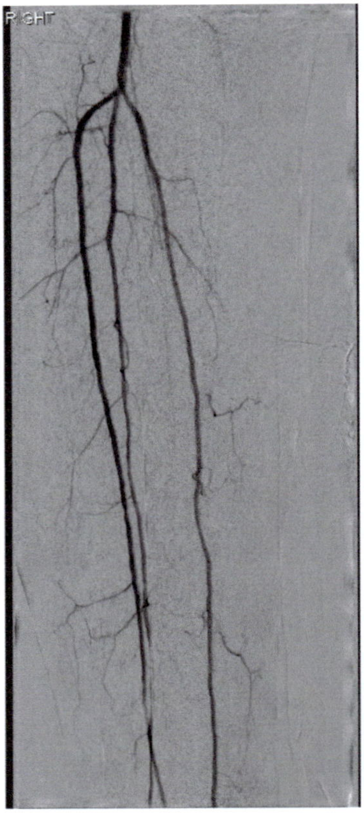

Fig. 2.2 Digital subtraction angiography (DSA) showing popliteal artery trifurcation with short segment occlusion of the distal peroneal artery

The genicular anastomosis has a superficial and deep network. The genicular anastomosis and collateral network in patients with popliteal artery occlusive disease are much less robust compared to the anastomosis of the brachial artery around the elbow.

The Anterior Tibial Artery

Near its origin, it passes through the superior part of the interosseous membrane to the front of the leg medial to the neck of the fibula. It descends in front of the interosseous membrane and below the malleoli and continues as the dorsalis pedis (DP) artery in the dorsum of the foot [1] (Fig. 2.3).

Variations The vessel may be smaller than average and may even be absent and replaced by the perforating branches of the PTA or a perforating branch of the peroneal artery. High origin of anterior tibial artery has been reported in 1.9%–4.2% of cases based on cadaveric and autopsy studies (Fig. 2.4). It then passes beneath (anterior) to the popliteus muscle [1].

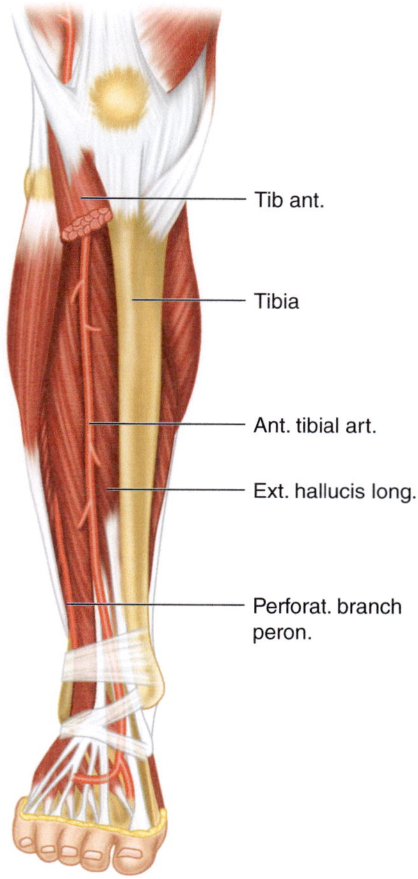

Fig. 2.3 Anatomy of the anterior tibial artery and dorsalis pedis artery

The dorsalis pedis artery is a continuation of the ATA distal to the ankle joint, and it follows along the tibial side of the dorsum of the foot to the proximal end of the first dorsal interosseous muscle to complete the plantar arch (Fig. 2.3).

The posterior tibial artery begins at the lower border of the popliteus and then courses downward and medially on the back of the leg. At the ankle, it is midway between the medial malleolus and medial tubercle of the calcaneus (Fig. 2.5).

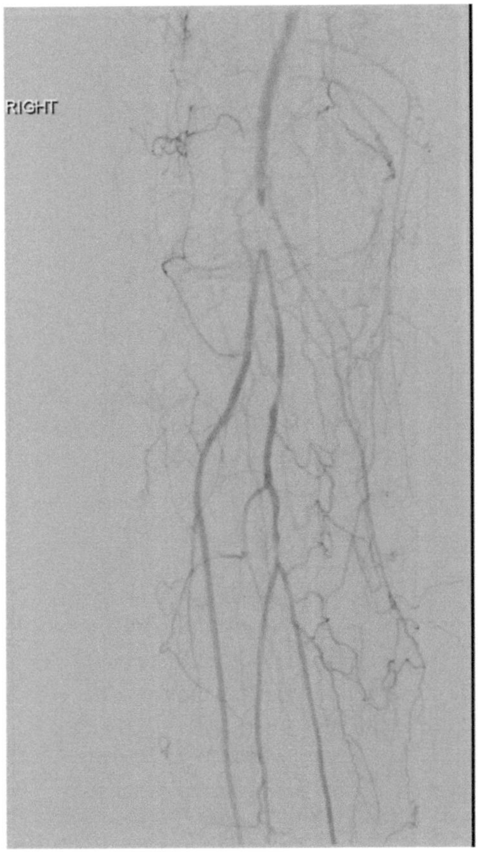

Fig. 2.4 Arteriogram showing a high origin of the anterior tibial artery just above the knee joint with associated short segment occlusion of the popliteal artery above the knee

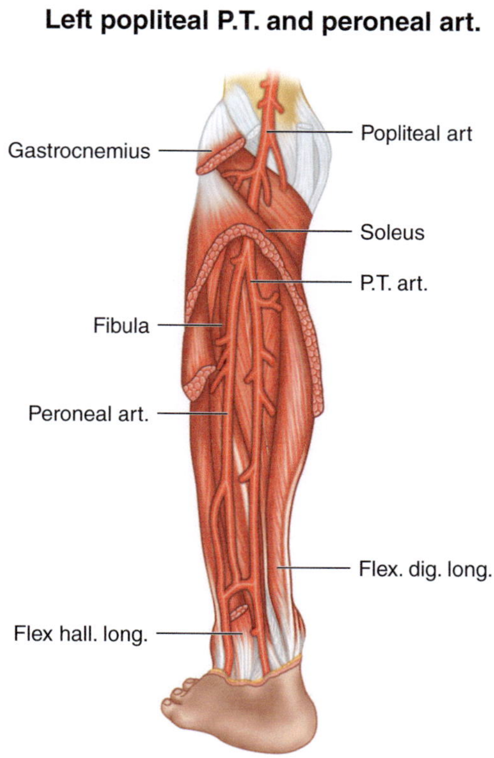

Fig. 2.5 Anatomy of the left popliteal artery, posterior artery, and peroneal artery

The Peroneal Artery

The peroneal artery arises from the PTA, 2.5 cm below the lower border of the popliteus, and it then courses obliquely toward the fibula and descends along its medial crest in a fibrous canal between the tibialis posterior and flexor hallucis longus or in the substance of the flexor hallucis longus. It then divides into calcaneal branches. The proximal segment of the peroneal artery is covered by soleus and deep transverse fascia. The distal portion is overlapped by flexor hallucis longus [1].

Variations The peroneal artery may arise from the tibial peroneal trunk more proximal than usual or may even arise from the popliteal artery. In some patients, the peroneal artery is large and either joins or reinforces PTA.

Veins There are two sets of veins in the lower extremity (LE): superficial and deep. The superficial veins course through the superficial fascia under the skin. The deep veins accompany the corresponding arteries. Both the superficial and deep veins have valves, which are more numerous in the deep venous system than in the superficial veins.

The Superficial Veins of the LE The main superficial veins are the great and small saphenous veins. The great (long) saphenous veins (GSV), the longest in the body, begins as the medial margin vein of the foot and terminates into the femoral vein approximately 2.5–3 cm below the inguinal ligament. It ascends in front of the medial malleolus for 2.5–3 cm and crosses the lower part of the medial surface of the tibia obliquely coursing along the medial border, about 1 cm posteriorly. It then ascends upward, posterior and medial to the medial condyles of the tibia and the femur, coursing along the medial side of the thigh and passing through the fossa ovalis to join the femoral vein [1].

In the thigh, it is accompanied by branches of the medial femoral cutaneous nerve; at the knee, by a branch of the descending genicular artery; and in the lower leg and foot, by the saphenous nerve which lies anterior to the vein. The great saphenous vein may be duplicated below the knee. There are 10–20 valves in the GSV, which are more numerous below the knee. Just before it pierces through the fossa ovalis, it is joined by the superficial epigastric, superficial external iliac, and superficial external pudendal vein [1].

The deep veins of the LE accompany the arteries [1].

The PT veins accompany the PTA. They receive veins from the soleus venous plexus, the superficial veins of the leg, and the peroneal veins.

The AT veins accompany the ATA. They leave the front of the leg by passing between the tibia and fibula through the proximal portion of the interosseous membrane of the leg and unite with the PT veins to form the popliteal vein [1].

The popliteal vein ascends through the popliteal fossa to the hiatus magnus where it becomes the femoral vein. Popliteal vein has three to five valves [1].

The femoral vein accompanies the SFA and ascends to the level of the inguinal ligament; it then becomes the external iliac vein. There are four to five valves in the superficial femoral vein (SFV), the most constant being just below the entrance of the profunda femoris vein. The femoral vein has a valve below the inguinal ligament [1].

The profunda femoris vein is anterior to the corresponding artery and receives tributaries corresponding to the muscular and perforating veins of that artery and, through these, establishes communications with the popliteal vein [1].

Lymphatics The superficial lymph vessels begin in the plexus of the lymphatics underneath the skin collecting vessels and leave the foot in a medial set, following the GSV and a lateral set and following the small saphenous vein. The lymphatic vessels of the medial group are larger and are greater in number than those of the lateral group; they ascend on the medial side of the dorsum of the foot and course along with GSV into the groin where they end in the inferior group of the superficial inguinal nodes; the vessels of the lateral group begin on the lateral side of the dorsum of the foot. Some cross the anterior aspect of the leg to join the vessels of the medial group and reach the lower group of the superficial inguinal lymph nodes; others go along with the small (lesser) saphenous vein and end in the popliteal lymph nodes [1].

Lymphatic drainage of the deeper tissues of the lower extremity: The deep lymph vessels accompany the main vasculature of the LE such as the AT, PT, peroneal, popliteal, and femoral sets. The deep vessels of the foot and leg may terminate in the popliteal nodes, but those from the thigh end directly in the deep group of inguinal lymph nodes [1].

Reference

1. Standring S. Gray's anatomy e-book: Gray's anatomy e-book. Amsterdam: Elsevier Health Sciences; 2021.

3 Duplex Sonography of Lower Extremity Aneurysmal Disease

Duplex sonography consists of a two-dimensional B-mode imaging system, a pulsed Doppler flow detector, and a spectrum analyzer. Transducer frequencies of approximately 3 MHz are most suitable for evaluating the abdominal vessels in average-sized adults, whereas a 5 MHz transducer can be used for thin individuals. Examination of the superficially located arteries in the lower extremities is generally performed with 5–7.5, or 10 MHz transducers [1]. The highest frequency head that provides adequate depth penetration should be selected. Color Doppler instruments combine standard duplex technology with a real-time color display of blood flow and flow abnormalities caused by arterial pathology. Color-duplex imaging is not a replacement for conventional duplex ultrasonography with spectral waveform analysis, as the latter remains the mainstay of duplex diagnostic information. Color-duplex ultrasound is readily available, noninvasive, cost-effective, and highly accurate; it can identify the diameter of the aneurysm, the presence or absence of intraluminal thrombus, and the anatomy of inflow and outflow arteries. The Doppler component can identify areas of associated stenosis, occlusion, existence of any arteriovenous connections, associated venous thrombosis, or venous compression if present [1]. The differentiation between true and pseudoaneurysms can be easily confirmed by color-duplex ultrasound including any hematoma overlying the vessels.

A true aneurysm has a circumferential dilation of the lumen of the vessel and is more commonly fusiform and rarely saccular. Aneurysms in the extremities tend to be fusiform. Arterial aneurysms in the lower extremity have associated intraluminal thrombus with potential risk of embolic occlusion of the distal arteries. Rupture of a peripheral artery aneurysm is relatively uncommon.

In contrast, pseudoaneurysms occur due to an injury to the vessel wall with a defect in all three layers of the vessel wall resulting in leakage of blood into the surrounding tissues, while the underlying vessel is of normal caliber. Color Doppler imaging can determine whether there is a "to-and-fro" arterial flow signal from the defect in the vessel, which is the so-called neck of the pseudoaneurysm. The

S. S. Hans, *Contemporary Management of Lower Extremity Aneurysmal Disease*,
https://doi.org/10.1007/978-3-032-00159-7_3

proximal native artery has a lower resistance spectral waveform compared to the artery distal to the pseudoaneurysm.

Aneurysms involving the arteries of the lower extremity (LE) are second in frequency of occurrence only to the aneurysms of the intrarenal aorta and iliac artery aneurysms. Most aneurysms in the femoral, popliteal, and infrapopliteal segments are degenerative in etiology, and pseudoaneurysms may occur following coronary or peripheral interventions using femoral artery access.

True femoral artery aneurysms occur far more commonly in men than in women at a ratio of 10:1, with associated aortic aneurysms in 62% of patients, iliac artery aneurysms in 60% of patients, and contralateral lower extremity (femoral and popliteal) aneurysms in 24% of patients.

Femoral Aneurysms: Clinical Presentation and Diagnosis

True aneurysms of the CFA commonly present as asymptomatic pulsatile mass in the groin, and the patient should be evaluated by color-duplex flow imaging (Figs. 3.1 and 3.2).

Femoral pseudoaneurysms are also pulsatile with local tenderness, bruising, and ecchymosis of the overlying skin. Audible bruit is often present due the "to-and-fro" movement of the blood from the artery into the soft tissues. Femoral anastomotic aneurysms following aortofemoral graft reconstruction are far more common than true femoral artery aneurysms and should be confirmed by duplex-color imaging.

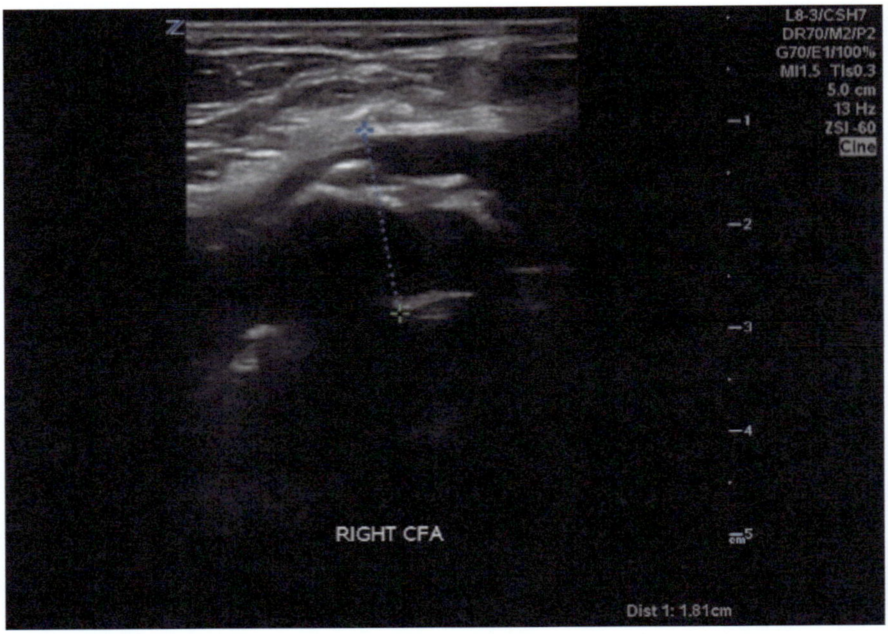

Fig. 3.1 Color-duplex imaging showing the right common femoral artery aneurysm

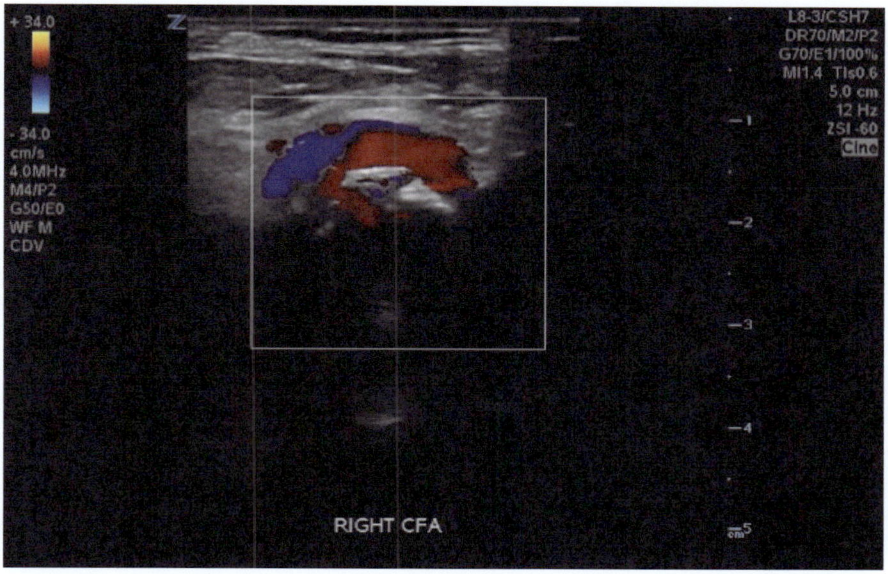

Fig. 3.2 Duplex imaging of the right common femoral artery aneurysm

Popliteal Artery Aneurysms: Clinical Presentation and Diagnosis

Popliteal aneurysms are often palpable in the popliteal fossa as a prominent pulse or as a pulsatile mass. Occasionally, popliteal artery aneurysm is detected incidentally during lower extremity venous imaging for suspected venous disease [2]. In some patients, popliteal aneurysm may be present with acute thrombosis, often resulting in acute ischemia. Color-duplex sonographic findings of popliteal artery aneurysm should routinely show the maximum diameter of the aneurysm, proximal extent of the aneurysm, distal extent of the aneurysm, and the presence of intraluminal thrombus (Figs. 3.3 and 3.4). In patients with acute ischemia due to thrombosed popliteal aneurysm, no color flow is detectable in the aneurysm sac. It has been reported that the average thrombus burden of 60% was significantly smaller in nonoperative popliteal artery aneurysms, as compared to 75% (IQR 58–89) in operative popliteal aneurysms ($p < 0.01$) [3]. Calculating a ratio between the thrombus size and patent channel overall percentage, the thrombus burden was larger in popliteal artery aneurysms of those who underwent operative interventions as compared to popliteal artery aneurysms managed nonoperatively [3]. Color-duplex sonography is extremely useful for follow-up evaluation of endovascular repair of popliteal aneurysms (Figs. 3.5, 3.6, and 3.7).

Infrapopliteal aneurysms are rarely palpable but may be present with pain or discomfort in the distal portion of the LE. Duplex ultrasound (DUS) with a 5–7 MHz transducer is the initial imaging study of choice as it can image both superficial and

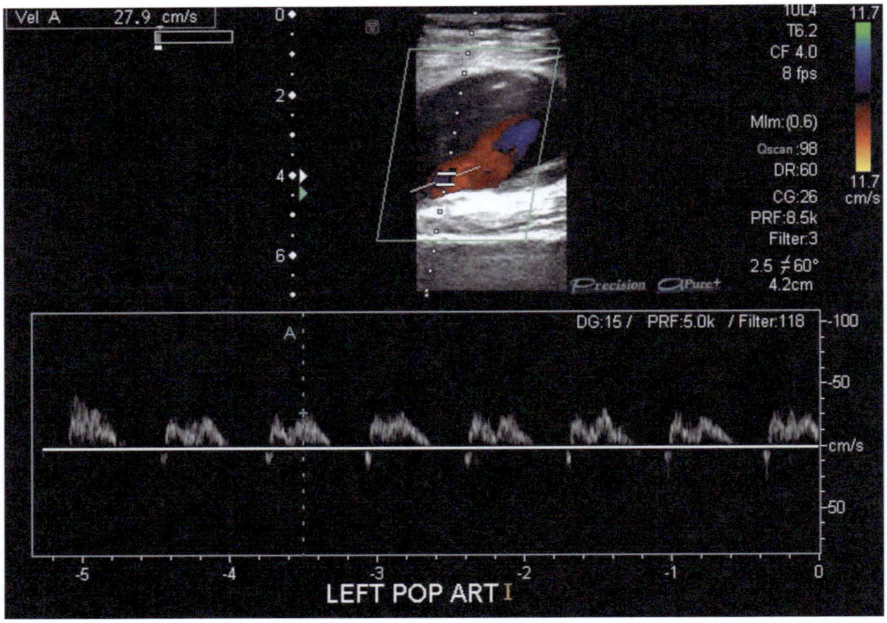

Fig. 3.3 Color-duplex imaging left popliteal artery aneurysm

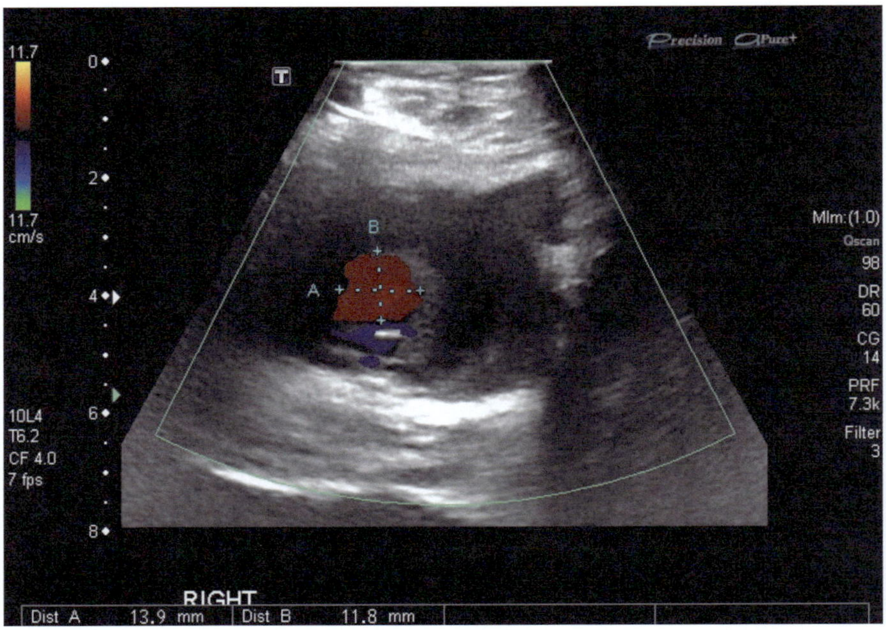

Fig. 3.4 Color Doppler imaging of the right popliteal artery aneurysm

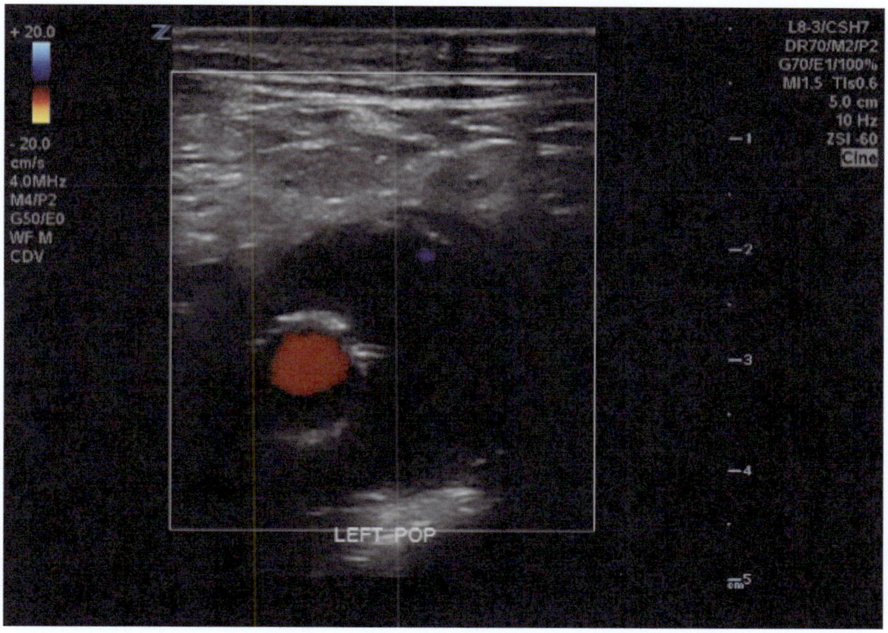

Fig. 3.5 Color-duplex imaging of the popliteal artery aneurysm with thrombus

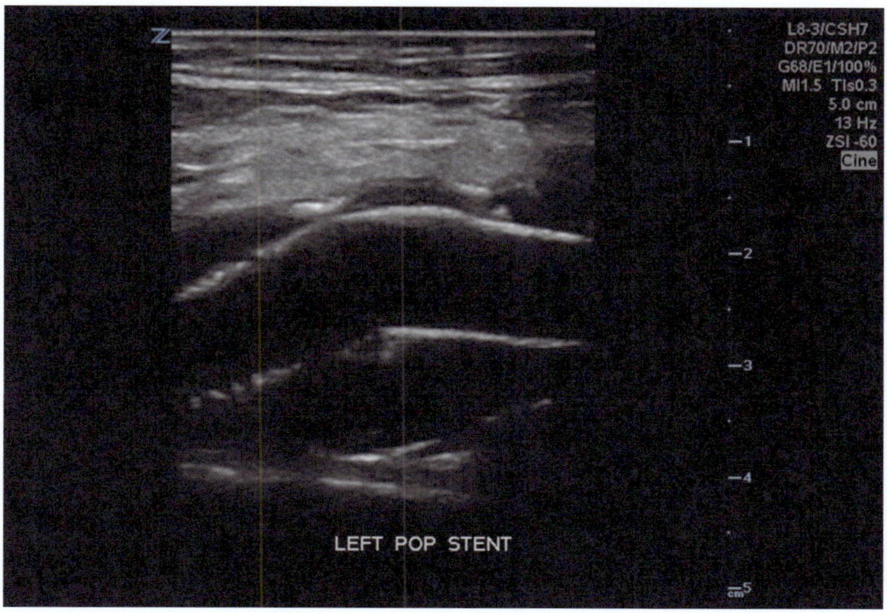

Fig. 3.6 Duplex imaging following the exclusion of the left popliteal aneurysm with endograft placement

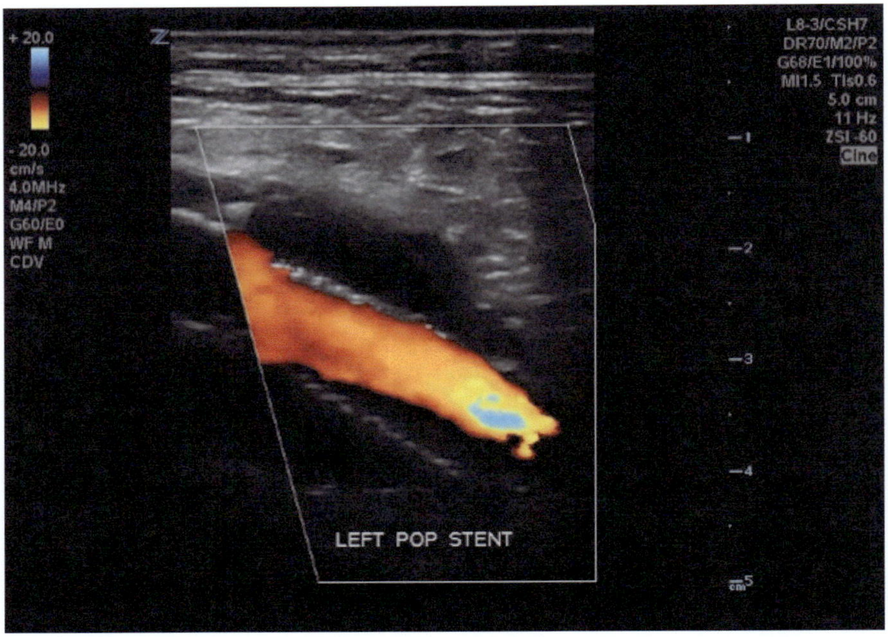

Fig. 3.7 Color-duplex imaging following the exclusion of the left popliteal aneurysm with endograft placement

deep vessels. The sensitivity and specificity of DUS is 94% and 97%, respectively, for the diagnosis of pseudoaneurysm [1]. A complete DUS should not only provide measurement of a maximal diameter of the vessel but also define the proximal and distal extent of the aneurysm. This information is important for the planning treatment of the aneurysms using endovascular or open repair. Infrapopliteal aneurysms are difficult to diagnose by clinical exam or DUS.

Invited Commentary

Anahita Dua, MD, MS, MBA

Duplex sonography stands as one of the pillars of diagnosis and evaluation of lower extremity aneurysms. While CT-angiogram provides an overall view of the aneurysmal anatomy, it is the ultrasound that provides key information including flow dynamics and thrombus burden, both crucial pieces of information when it comes to interventional decision-making. Ultrasonography specifically provides information regarding aneurysmal size, which has historically been the primary factor in operative planning.

On average, aneurysms >2 cm in the femoral-popliteal segment support operative management primarily in the popliteal segment as this can be associated with embolus; this complication is highly associated with amputation and as such is one of the more morbid complications associated with lower extremity aneurysms. Therefore, as stated in the chapter, when ultrasound identified thrombus burden, intervention is favored, but up until recently, the quantitative thrombus burden associated with embolus had never been quantified. Dua and colleagues [4] evaluated 470 popliteal aneurysms in 331 patients with duplex ultrasonography in a retrospective cross-sectional cohort study and found that in a multivariate analysis, higher percent thrombus was significantly associated with symptomatic aneurysms (RRR 15.2; CI 2.69–72.3; $P < 0.01$) and popliteal aneurysms with an acutely limb threatening event (RRR 17.9; CI 3.76–85.0; $P < 0.01$) [4]. All other anatomic characteristics were not associated with symptom status including size. This data supports the aggressive use of duplex sonography in evaluating lower extremity aneurysms. Unfortunately, a manuscript published by this group also assessed duplex reports of lower extremity aneurysm for inclusion of information pertinent to operative decision-making and timing of surveillance and found in a multi-institutional retrospective study, that aneurysms are often not followed at intervals recommended by the Society for Vascular Surgery guidelines and did not include all measurements necessary for clinical decision-making [3]. They concluded that there should be standardization of DUS protocols performed by all noninvasive vascular laboratories to ensure completeness of DUS images and inclusion of characteristics pertinent to clinical decision-making in radiology reports [3].

Overall, duplex sonography for aneurysm is a vital part of decision-making and can provide key information, but standardizing how we approach these patients on a national level is the key to optimally using this excellent technology.

References

1. Jacobowitz GR. Color duplex ultrasound for diagnosis of peripheral artery aneurysms (lower and upper extremity). In: AbuRahma AF, Perler BA, editors. Noninvasive vascular diagnosis: a practical textbook for clinicians. Cham: Springer International Publishing; 2022. p. 1–13.
2. Dalsing MC, Gonzalez AA, Maijub JG, et al. Prevalence and associations of incidental non-venous duplex findings discovered during lower extremity venous imaging. J Vasc Surg Venous Lymphat Disord. 2021;9(1):200–8. https://doi.org/10.1016/j.jvsv.2020.06.013. Epub 20200627. PubMed PMID: 32599309.
3. Bellomo TR, Goudot G, Gaston B, Lella S, Jessula S, Sumetsky N, Beardsley J, Patel S, Fischetti C, Zacharias N, Dua A, et al. Popliteal artery aneurysm ultrasound criteria for reporting characteristics. Vasc Med. 2024;29(1):58–63. https://doi.org/10.1177/1358863x231215781. Epub 20231222. PubMed PMID: 38131163.
4. Bellomo TR, Goudot G, Lella SK, Gaston B, Sumetsky N, Patel S, Zacharias N, Dua A. Percent thrombus predicts popliteal artery aneurysm related limb threatening events. Ann Surg. 2024; https://doi.org/10.1097/SLA.0000000000006352. Online ahead of print. PMID: 38771946.

MRA and CT Angiography of Lower Extremity Aneurysmal Disease

4

Computed tomography angiography (CTA) is an effective noninvasive imaging modality that provides the vascular specialist and the radiologist with a rapid, widely available, and accurate means to diagnose or confirm the diagnosis of femoral, popliteal, and infrapopliteal artery aneurysms. It also helps in planning the management of lower extremity aneurysmal disease. As compared to digital subtraction angiography, CTA is significantly less expensive and less invasive and allows for three-dimensional visualization from multiple angles and directions [1]. Prior to imaging with CTA, the potential nephrotoxic effects of iodinated contrast media should be evaluated. In patients with normal renal function, CTA has been shown to be safe with no evidence of deterioration of renal function (Glomerular filtration rate (GFR)).

Three-dimensional post-processing with maximum intensity projection (MIP), multiplanar reformatted, 3D virtual reality (VR) images and shaded surface displays can be used to augment analysis of the reconstructed cross-sectional axial images. Three phases of imaging are usually performed: pre-contrast imaging, arterial phase imaging, and venous (delayed) phase imaging. Arterial phase imaging is performed typically with either a fixed scan delay or bolus tracking [1]. A fixed scan delay of 40 s enables imaging to automatically commence after the delay. Meanwhile, bolus tracking relies on achieving a preferred attenuation (usually 100–120 Hounsfield units) within the area of interest such as infrarenal aorta, and imaging is initiated after a fixed time. Typically, 100 cc of iodinated contrast is used, but the quantity may be increased in order to image a larger patient or diminished if the patient is scanned on a newer equipment with a faster speed table [1]. Lowering the x-ray tube voltage and increasing the pitch with a helical CT scan decrease the radiation exposure. Three-dimensional post-processing with MIP, multiplanar reformatted, 3D CTA images and shaded surface displays can be used to augment

S. S. Hans, *Contemporary Management of Lower Extremity Aneurysmal Disease*,
https://doi.org/10.1007/978-3-032-00159-7_4

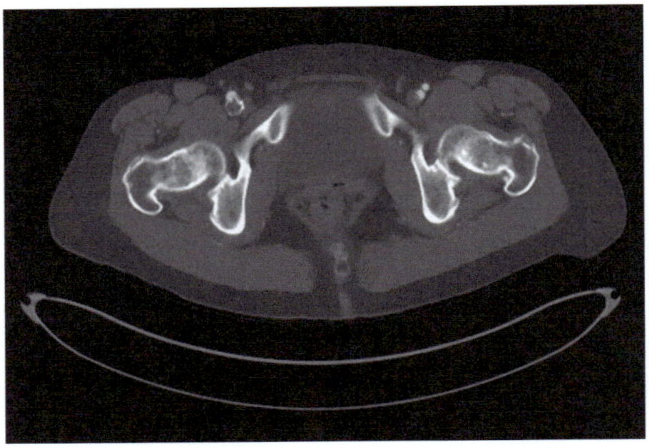

Fig. 4.1 CTA showing the right common femoral artery aneurysm

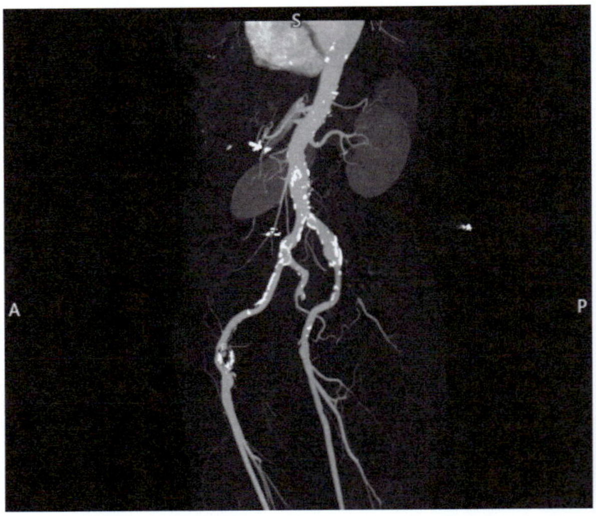

Fig. 4.2 CTA showing MIP images of the right common femoral artery aneurysm

the analysis of the reconstructed cross-sectional axial images (Figs. 4.1 and 4.2). Imaging the entire course of the vessel in a single plane/centerline is useful in evaluating vascular anatomy and endograft repair or open arterial reconstruction. In most instances, popliteal aneurysms have a significant amount of intraluminal thrombus (Fig. 4.3).

In patients with severe renal dysfunction (GFR <30 mL/min/1.73 m^2), CTA should be avoided in favor of MRA or CO_2 angiography. In patients with GFR between 30–40 prehydration and post-hydration for 12 h with intravenous NS infusion (100 cc per hour), reduction in the volume has shown to reduce the incidence of contrast-induced nephropathy. The use of nonionic iso-osmolar contrast is associated with the lowest risk of contrast-induced nephropathy.

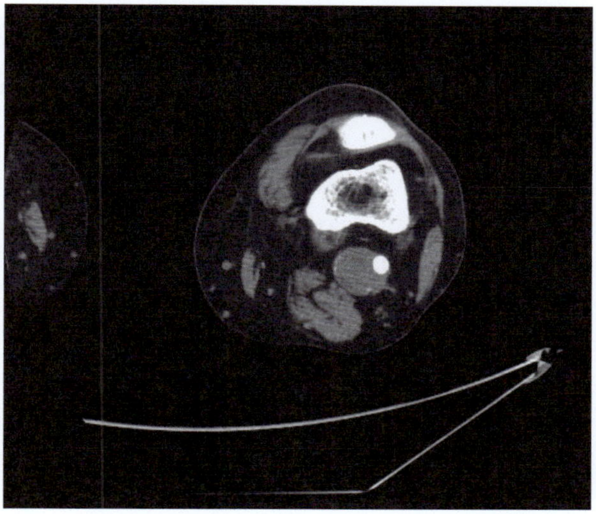

Fig. 4.3 CTA showing the popliteal aneurysm with significant amount of intraluminal thrombus

Mean Diameters of the Normal Aorta and the Lower Extremity Arteries in Adults

Vessel	Range (Mean) mm
Infra-renal aorta	19.9–23.9 (16.6–21.6)
Common iliac	11.7–12.3 (9.7–10.2)
Common femoral	7.9–8.5
SFA	6–6.3
Popliteal	5.9–6.2
PT arterial	2.0–2.2

CTA examination of patients with femoral artery and popliteal artery aneurysms should include the aortic and pelvic vasculature to diagnose additional aneurysms if present. CTA has a better spatial resolution than MRA.

MRA is the only vascular imaging technique that can be performed without the use of contrast media, a technique referred to as time-of-flight (TOF) MRA. In contrast to routine MRI, TOF MRA expresses a signal from stationary tissues instead of using the movement of blood in the lumen of the blood vessels to create a signal referred to as flow-related enhancement. In order to isolate the flow in arteries, venous flow enhancement is excluded by using saturation bands above the imaging volume, thus saturating the flow from the cranial to caudal direction. TOF MRA can be performed using both 2D and 3D acquisition modes. Some advantages of the 2D mode include shorter imaging time, better sensitivity to slow flow, and the ability to visualize long segments of blood vessels. The disadvantages include decrease sensitivity to in-plane flow and decreased spatial resolution. A stair-step artifact worsened by patient motion can be seen. Three-dimensional TOF MRA (3D TOF MRA) is more commonly used to evaluate the head and the circle of Willis and a smaller area where imaging is needed [2]; in addition, 3D TOF MRA has superior resolution. Disadvantages include insensitivity to slow flow and longer acquisition time. Contrast-enhanced MRA (CE-MRA) relies on an intravascular contrast agent to directly generate a signal within the vessel lumen. CE MRA can acquire the same imaging volume in a shorter period using a

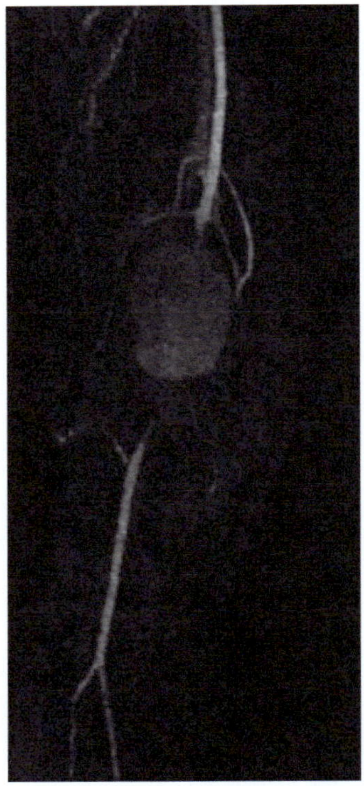

Fig. 4.4 MRA showing the right popliteal aneurysm

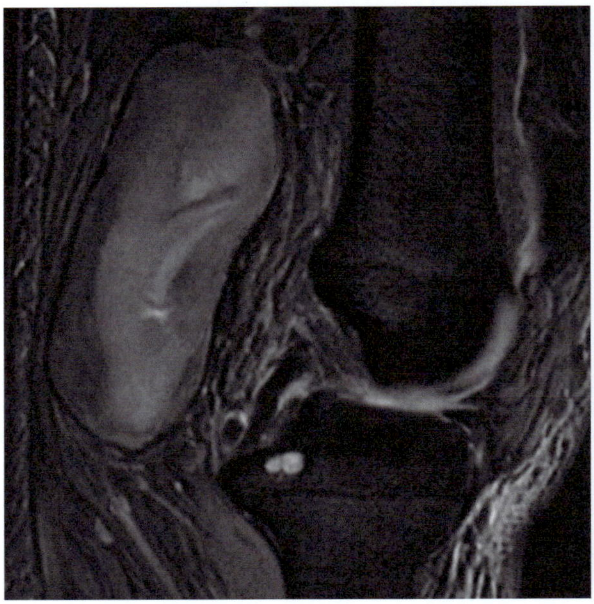

Fig. 4.5 Coronal view MRA showing the right popliteal aneurysm

single-breath-hold for imaging; a CE MRA with larger field of view is also acquired in the coronal plane. CE MRA is more accurate than TOF MRA in the settings of slow flow or high-grade stenosis, which can be overestimated with TOF MRA (Figs. 4.4 and 4.5). Phase-contrast MRA, a non-contrast imaging technique, is more often used for MR venography. Typically, MRA is performed using a hybrid approach combining time-resolved MRA (TR-MRA) of the calves with first-pass MRA (FP-MRA) of the abdomen, pelvis, and thighs [3]. Conventional agents are not retained within the vascular space; thus, their use necessitates fast imaging to provide the required vessel/tissue contrast which limits spatial resolution. In fact, poor spatial resolution has been one of the drawbacks of MRA compared to CTA, which is usually preferable for visualization of the infrapopliteal vessels [3].

Gadofosveset trisodium can be used for image enhancement and has an extended half-life of up to 60 min. This extended period of enhancement allows acquisition of images with increased spatial resolution during the equilibrium phase of circulation (5–10 min after contrast injection), with simultaneous visualization of both arteries and veins [3].

The potential drawbacks of using the equilibrium phase images with blood pool contrast agents include motion artifacts due to the extended scanning time and venous signals, which may diminish the visualization of the small arteries.

Invited Commentary

Milan V. Pantelic, MD, MSE, FACR

In the years since the advent of helical scan technology, CT has risen to a preeminent role in noninvasive vascular imaging, complimenting ultrasound with its speed, ubiquitous access, spatial resolution, and breadth of anatomic coverage. Subsequent innovations incorporating large-field or dual-source detector systems have further increased both the speed and spatial resolution of CTA acquisitions, while reducing patient radiation exposure and required contrast volumes. Current advances, including photon-counting detectors which can significantly increase the achievable image resolution and spectral imaging which further augments image contrast and can separate iodine (intravascular contrast) from calcium and other tissues, are gradually moving into the mainstream and will further cement CT as a "Swiss Army knife" in vascular imaging.

While MRI is a tremendously powerful tool for diagnosis, it remains a second-line imaging modality in the setting of peripheral vascular disease; despite the benefits of nonionizing radiation, potential avoidance of intravenous contrast, and lack of significant nephrotoxicity of IV contrast agents, MRI is of more limited availability, requires greater imaging time and patient cooperation, and necessitates higher-end systems with greater radiologist expertise to deploy the most advanced MR imaging sequences. The referring vascular care specialist may have less familiarity and comfort with MRA imaging, further limiting its utilization in routine practice.

In comparison to conventional 2D time-of-flight sequences, newer MR imaging techniques incorporating inflow preparation or sensitization, dynamic acquisition, and improved background suppression have significantly improved non-contrast peripheral vascular imaging. Current contrast-enhanced MRA acquisitions can approach conventional CT for in-plane spatial resolution, are much less limited by calcifications, and use time-resolved techniques to provide dynamic inflow information analogous to catheter angiography. Furthermore, these techniques can be combined in ways that allow for multiple contrast administrations, combinations of non-contrast and contrast-enhanced imaging, and imaging incorporating positional changes or stress maneuvers. Concomitant MR imaging of the blood vessel wall can yield further diagnostic information, for example, in distinguishing inflammatory arteritides from atherosclerotic or other vessel wall disease.

While MRA with the blood pool contrast agent gadofosveset trisodium allowed both conventional dynamic or bolus-chase MRA, and subsequent high-resolution imaging of steady-state vascular enhancement of the arteries and veins at equivalent spatial resolution to CT, this agent is no longer available. Steady-state vascular enhancement MRA can be achieved, albeit at considerably lower efficiency, with gadobenate dimeglumine, a linear gadolinium-chelate contrast agent, though it is rarely employed for this purpose due to its much weaker plasma protein binding and resultant lower-level enhancement. Both dynamic and steady-state MRA of the central and peripheral vasculature can be achieved with off-label use of intravenous ultrasmall superparamagnetic iron oxide (USPIO) particle preparation (ferumoxytol), a pharmaceutical initially designed as a blood pool MR contrast agent, but currently marketed and approved for parenteral iron supplementation. Ferumoxytol MRA is useful when there are contraindications to iodinated contrast and gadolinium-chelate contrast, including in cases of renal insufficiency, contrast allergy, and congenital heart and other pediatric populations.

Although contrast-enhanced CTA remains the noninvasive mainstay in imaging of peripheral arterial disease, MRA has significant advantages in certain clinical contexts. Consultation between the vascular care specialist and radiologist is essential in more complex cases, to ensure optimal use of advanced MR imaging for patient benefit.

References

1. Ofer A, Nitecki SS, Linn S, et al. Multidetector CT angiography of peripheral vascular disease: a prospective comparison with intraarterial digital subtraction angiography. AJR Am J Roentgenol. 2003;180(3):719–24. https://doi.org/10.2214/ajr.180.3.1800719. PubMed PMID: 12591682.
2. Brott TG, Halperin JL, Abbara S, et al. 2011 ASA/ACCF/AHA/AANN/AANS/ACR/ASNR/CNS/SAIP/SCAI/SIR/SNIS/SVM/SVS guideline on the management of patients with extracranial carotid and vertebral artery disease: executive summary: a report of the American College of Cardiology Foundation/American Heart Association Task Force on Practice Guidelines, and the American Stroke Association, American Association of Neuroscience Nurses, American Association of Neurological Surgeons, American College of Radiology, American Society of Neuroradiology, Congress of Neurological Surgeons, Society of Atherosclerosis Imaging and Prevention, Society for Cardiovascular Angiography and Interventions, Society of Interventional Radiology, Society of NeuroInterventional Surgery, Society for Vascular Medicine, and Society for Vascular Surgery. J Am Coll Cardiol. 2011;57(8):1002–44. https://doi.org/10.1016/j.jacc.2010.11.005. Epub 20110201. PubMed PMID: 21288680.
3. Galizia MS, Ward E, Rodriguez H, et al. Improved characterization of popliteal aneurysms using gadofosveset-enhanced equilibrium phase magnetic resonance angiography. J Vasc Surg. 2013;57(3):837–41. https://doi.org/10.1016/j.jvs.2012.09.018. Epub 20130104. PubMed PMID: 23294506.
4. Campeau L. Percutaneous radial artery approach for coronary angiography. Cathet Cardiovasc Diagn. 1989;16:3–7.
5. Titano J. Safety and outcomes of transradial access in patients with international normalized radio 1.5 or above. J Vasc Interv Radiol. 2018;29(3):383–8.

Catheter-Based Arteriography for Evaluation of the Lower Extremity Aneurysmal Disease

5

In spite of the wide availability of color-duplex imaging, CTA, and MRA, diagnostic catheter arteriography remains extremely valuable for the diagnosis and assessment of peripheral arterial disease and for its applicability to therapeutic interventions such as thrombolytic therapy, endograft deployment, and open arterial reconstruction of the lower extremity for aneurysmal disease. At present, the standard for contrast arteriography of the lower extremity is intra-arterial DSA in place of previously used conventional film-screen arteriography. Film-screen arteriography uses a cut sheet of film stacked or placed in a roll within a delivery magazine or cassette called a rapid-fire film changer; rapid-fire film changers carry between 20 and 30 14 × 14 inch films. Conventional arteriography is based on image acquisition after contrast media injection, and the final image includes blood vessels, bones, and other tissues. This superimposition of nonvascular structures makes it difficult to get an accurate visualization of the blood vessels. In order to obtain the best visualization of vascular structures, a pre-contrast image (mask image) is acquired as a first step and is digitally subtracted from the post-contrast images after removal of distracting structures, thus enabling high-quality arteriograms. With DSA, small caliber vessels can be visualized with the use of a much smaller volume of contrast medium [1].

Preprocedure evaluation Renal function (blood urea nitrogen (BUN), creatinine, GFR) should be obtained in all patients as iodinated contrast media are nephrotoxic. In patients with impaired renal function, hydration with administration of 0.9 normal saline (NS) at the rate of 100 cc per hour for 12 h prior to arteriography and 12 h after arteriography, the use of smaller volume of contrast media, and the use of diluted contrast media can reduce the incidence of contrast-induced nephropathy. Patients allergic to iodine or with a history of prior adverse reaction to iodinated contrast media should be premedicated with steroids and antihistamines. A severe

S. S. Hans, *Contemporary Management of Lower Extremity Aneurysmal Disease*,
https://doi.org/10.1007/978-3-032-00159-7_5

anaphylactic reaction to iodine has been reported in 0.04% of patients receiving a nonionic contrast agent. Risk factors associated with these reactions include female gender, asthma, and previous reactions to contrast media. An allergy to seafood or fish is not associated with a greater incidence of reaction to contrast media. The mechanism of these reactions is most often due to a direct effect on basophil or mast cell and not due to iodine atoms. These cells release histamine and other mediators and then induce immediate hypersensitivity reaction (IHR) via IgE-mediated or non-IgE pathways, such as the complement system pathway [1].

Death from a contrast media reaction occurs in the order of 1–2 per 100,000 procedures. In patients with severe iodine allergy or renal dysfunction, alternative methods of evaluation such as MRA or the use of CO_2 in place of iodinated contrast agent should be considered for the evaluation of the lower extremity arterial system [1].

A. *Technique of Arteriography*

For the evaluation of lower extremity aneurysms (femoral, popliteal, and infrapopliteal), contralateral femoral access is preferred. In patients with prior aortic endografts and aortoiliac prosthetic grafts, left brachial access is preferable as passing the catheter over the acute angle of endograft or aortoiliac/femoral Dacron graft can be technically challenging. Femoral access is obtained using ultrasound with a micropuncture technique, followed by placement of a 5F sheath in the contralateral CFA; a 0.035" wire (Bentson or Starter guidewire) and an Omniflush catheter are advanced and positioned just superior to the renal arteries. The Omniflush catheter (or internal mammary artery catheter) is then brought caudally to the aortic bifurcation, and the contralateral common iliac and external iliac arteries are cannulated with the catheter advanced into the common femoral artery over the wire. A runoff study is obtained preferably using a pressure injector. Common femoral artery bifurcation is optimally visualized by an ipsilateral oblique position of the image intensifier. In order to obtain the optimal visualization of a thrombosed popliteal aneurysm and infrapopliteal arteries (runoff), a diagnostic catheter often needs to be advanced into the distal SFA (Figs. 5.1, 5.2, 5.3, and 5.4). Because of the presence of laminated thrombus in the aneurysmal wall, in most instances, therefore, arteriography is not useful in determining the exact size of the aneurysm.

The new angiography machines have automated sequences which set the frame speed and exposure time to different segments of the lower extremity arteries to be

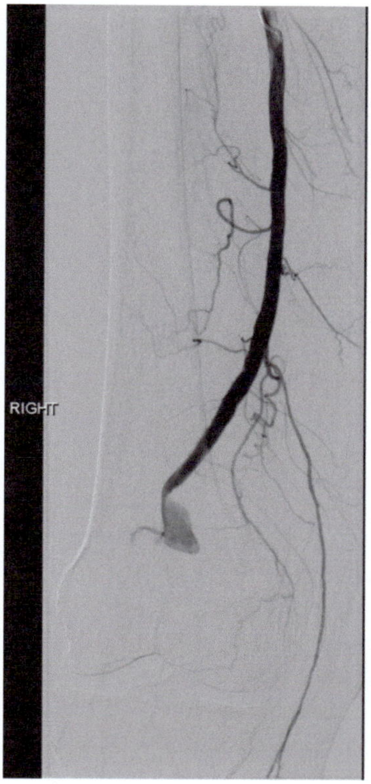

Fig. 5.1 Arteriogram showing the thrombosed right popliteal aneurysm

studied. Advanced computer processor power has made subtraction, pixel shifting, re-masking, or view tracing simple and feasible. The operator at the angiographic table can easily perform road mapping (superimposition) of the fluoroscopic image in a DSA image and the subtracted image referencing (fluoro save mode) collection; the magnification edge filters positioning of the table and the gantry angle can be changed by the operator to optimize visualization of the arteries. The introduction of high-resolution flat panel image intensifiers provides great quality-minimize parallax distortion. New flat panels have a large field of view that can cover large body segments, reduce the volume of contrast media, and reduce the radiation exposure to the patient and the operator [1].

To improve the visualization of infrapopliteal arteries, intravenous administration of nitroglycerine is useful in patients with acute thrombosis of popliteal aneurysm presenting with acute limb ischemia. The catheter for thrombolysis should be

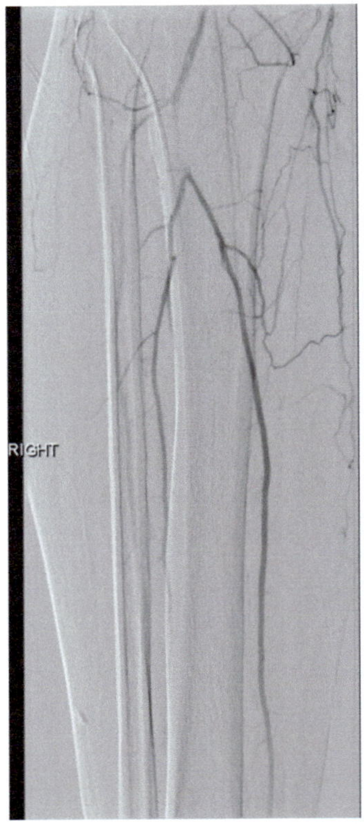

Fig. 5.2 Arteriogram showing two-vessel runoff with poor visualization of the tibioperoneal trunk

advanced into the distal popliteal artery in order to restore patency of infrapopliteal arteries prior to the arterial bypass for revascularization.

After the removal of the catheter and the wires, the femoral/brachial sheath is removed, and manual compression is performed for 5–10 min following access to obtain hemostasis. There has been increasing use of arterial closure devices during the last two decades to promote early ambulation and reduction in the time spent in the hospital after the procedure for femoral artery closure.

Fig. 5.4 (**a**) Arteriogram showing left popliteal aneurysm. (**b**) Arteriogram showing left popliteal artery aneurysm with three-vessel runoff

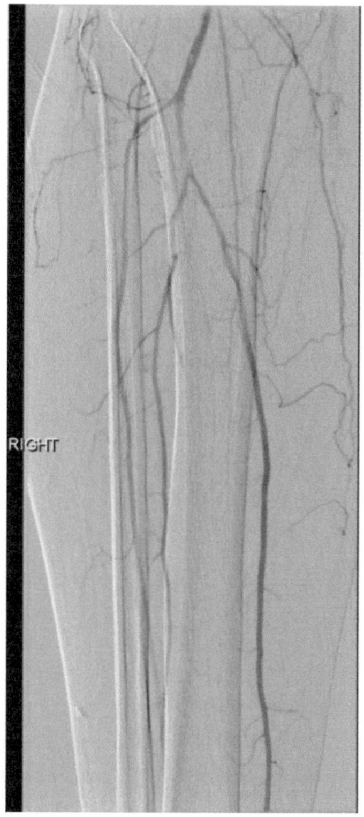

Fig. 5.3 Arteriogram showing retrograde filling of the tibioperoneal trunk via collaterals

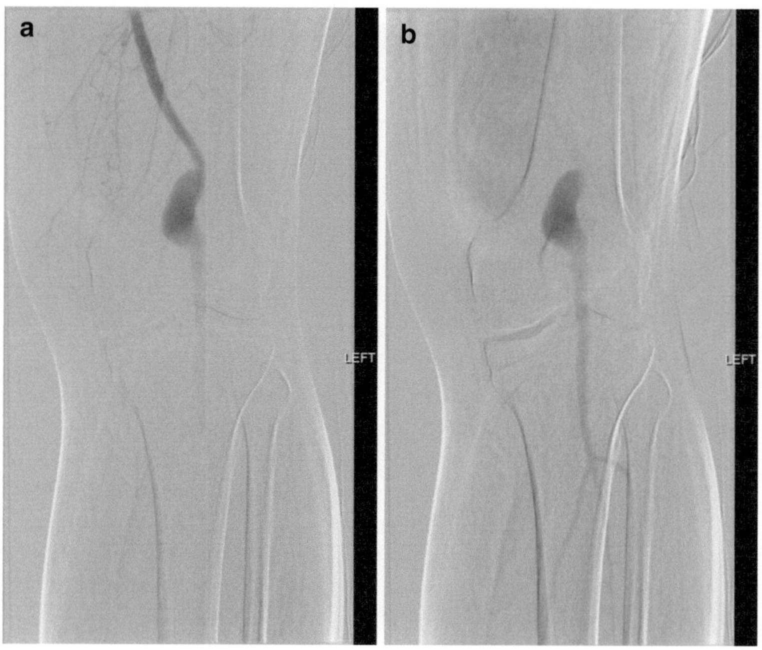

Complications

A. *Arterial Access-Related Complications*

Arteriography is well tolerated by most patients, with a low complication rate, but there is a risk of complications and even occasional mortality. The most common access-related complication is hematoma at the puncture site. A review of 34 articles during the past 10 years shows that for both diagnostic and therapeutic percutaneous interventions, using femoral access, complication rates, safety, and efficacy were comparable between vascular closure devices and manual compression [2]. Most groin hematomas are self-limiting, and the use of a larger sheath (from 5F to 11F) increases the risk of hematoma formation. A hematoma is usually detected immediately after sheath removal during manual compression at the site. Puncture cephalad to inguinal ligament results in an ineffective manual compression with the potential of retroperitoneal hemorrhage often necessitating surgical intervention. Other complications include dissection, thrombosis, and pseudoaneurysm formation.

B. *Risks Related to Contrast Media*

The use of iodinated contrast in patients with preexisting CKD (chronic kidney disease) (GFR < 45 mL/min/1.73 m^2) should be avoided. CO_2 angiography or MRA should be considered for such patients.

C. *Radiation Dose*

The use of DSA technique is associated with a high dose of radiation with its attendant risks. It is important to use post-processing imaging to improve DSA image quality and reduce the radiation dose. Important precautions include appropriate training in radiation safety, usage of the available dose reduction, quality of instruments/gear, and the lowest acceptable fluoroscopy rates. For reducing radiation exposure, magnification should be avoided if possible, as well as the usage of last image hold, recorded loops, and utilization of collimators.

Invited Commentary

Shehbaz Shaikh, MD

This chapter by Dr. Hans provides the reader with a well-written overview in performing catheter-based angiography of the lower extremity, as well as periprocedural management. Noninvasive vascular imaging such as ultrasound, CTA, and MRA may provide much information needed for appropriate treatment planning; however, digital subtraction angiography remains the gold standard.

The chapter discusses arteriography technique using common femoral artery access with brachial artery access reserved for patients with technically challenging anatomy, such as patients with prior aortoiliac endografts. Radial access is being increasingly used for diagnostic purposes and for intervention in patients with coronary and peripheral arterial disease. Radial access for coronary angiography was first described in 1989 and is currently popular amongst interventional cardiology and radiology labs [4]. The safety of radial access is well documented in the literature and is associated with low complication rates even in patients with an elevated INR [5]. Left radial access for peripheral interventions is achieved by placement of a specially designed 5F × 119 cm long hydrophilic sheath through which a 5F × 150 cm catheter is placed into the SFA. Following procedure completion, the sheath may be removed, and a commercially available wrist band with an inflatable balloon maintains hemostasis.

As technology continues to evolve, radial access equipment will likely expand to allow for even larger sheaths/catheters, or smaller profile balloons/stents will be developed. Vascular surgeons and interventionalists should be familiar with radial access as an alternative to brachial access in patients with challenging anatomy or for use as a primary access site.

References

1. Posa A, Tanzilli A, Barbieri P, et al. Digital subtraction angiography (DSA) technical and diagnostic aspects in the study of lower limb arteries. Radiation. 2022;2(4):376–86. https://doi.org/10.3390/radiation2040028. PubMed PMID.
2. Noori VJ, Eldrup-Jørgensen J. A systematic review of vascular closure devices for femoral artery puncture sites. J Vasc Surg. 2018;68(3):887–99. https://doi.org/10.1016/j.jvs.2018.05.019. Epub 20180629. PubMed PMID: 30146036.

Degenerative Femoral Artery Aneurysms

6

Degenerative femoral artery aneurysms are uncommon but have a significant clinical importance because of their potential to cause limb-threatening ischemia from acute thrombosis or distal embolization from the mural thrombus; the incidence of rupture of the aneurysm is relatively low. Most aneurysms of the lower extremities are degenerative in nature; on the other hand, pseudoaneurysms are the result of traumatic, anastomotic, and mycotic etiologies. Common risk factors for aneurysm formation include male gender, older age, smoking, and hypertension. In rare cases, connective tissue pathology such as Marfan syndrome may result in aneurysmal degeneration.

The reported incidence of degenerative femoral artery aneurysm is 5 patients per 100,000. From a study of 236 femoral artery aneurysms identified in 182 patients at eight institutions, the mean age was 72 years, with a male/female ratio of 16:1 [1]. Degenerative femoral artery aneurysms are more frequent in the common femoral artery CFA (57%), followed by superficial femoral artery SFA (26%) and profunda femoris artery (17%). Aneurysms that are limited to the CFA are classified as type I, while those involving the origin of profunda femoris artery are cited as type II because this distinction has important bearing on vascular reconstruction options. The incidence of synchronous aneurysms (mean 1.7 per patient) involving the aorta ($n = 133$), iliac arteries ($n = 107$), popliteal arteries ($n = 86$), and hypogastric arteries ($n = 56$) was reported in a series of 236 femoral artery aneurysms (2002–2012) from 48 institutions. The reported incidence of the contralateral CFA aneurysms are as follows: ($n = 34$), SFA ($n = 9$), and DFA (profunda $n = 2$).

Clinical presentation of degenerative CFA aneurysms varies from asymptomatic to severe lower extremity ischemia and occasional rupture of the aneurysm. The most common indicator for the repair of CFA aneurysms is the presence of an asymptomatic mass in 66% of patients, symptoms of intermittent claudication in 18%, local pain in 8%, nerve compression in 3%, and rupture in 2%, thus warranting intervention.

Diagnosis is usually made during the physical examination by the presence of a pulsatile groin mass upon palpation. As discussed in Chaps. 3, 4, and 5, imaging

S. S. Hans, *Contemporary Management of Lower Extremity Aneurysmal Disease*,
https://doi.org/10.1007/978-3-032-00159-7_6

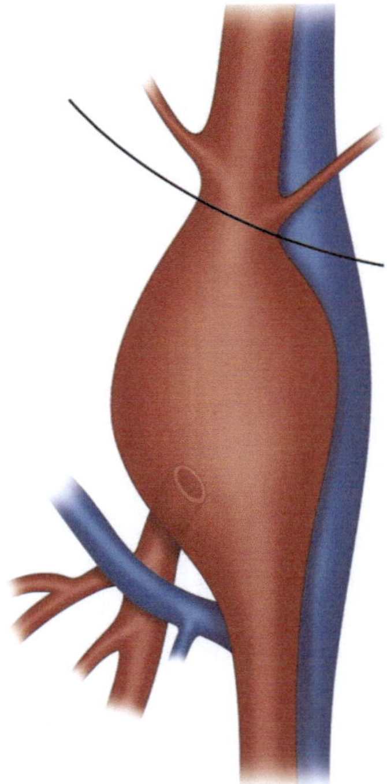

Fig. 6.1 Exposed right common femoral artery aneurysm. Vein crossing the origin of the deep (profunda) femoral artery

modalities such as color-duplex ultrasound, CTA, or MRA can confirm the diagnosis (Fig. 6.1). Catheter-based arteriography has a limited role in the diagnosis of FAA, as it only demonstrates the true lumen of an artery and may miss the diagnosis of an aneurysm and its size. The catheter-based arteriography visualizes the true lumen but not the exact size of the aneurysm with mural thrombus. Arteriography is useful in patients with associated occlusive disease and for operative planning.

Indications for treatment All symptomatic degenerative femoral artery aneurysms should be repaired. Previous studies have recommended surgical repair for common femoral artery aneurysms measuring greater than 2.5 cm in diameter even if asymptomatic. From the study of 236 femoral artery degenerative aneurysms, Lawrence et al. concluded that the repair criteria of asymptomatic femoral Artery Aneurysm (FAAs) should be changed to the size of 3.5 cm.

Preoperative planning Prospective cardiovascular risk assessment is important in nonemergent cases of FAAs given the advanced age and multiple comorbidities in this patient population. Besides appropriate imaging studies, bilateral lower extremity arterial Doppler study with segmental pressure, Ankle-brachial index (ABI), and toe-brachial index should be obtained.

Repair Although few case reports of endovascular repair in extremely high-risk patients have been described, almost all patients with FAA need open repair with replacement of aneurysmal segment with an interposition synthetic graft (Dacron or polytetrafluoroethylene (PTFE)). The autologous vein as a conduit for an interposition graft is not recommended except in mycotic aneurysms. The synthetic graft has a similar size with that of the common femoral artery and with satisfactory patency rates because the required length of the graft is relatively short.

General or regional (epidural) anesthesia is preferable during the repair. The procedure can be performed under a local anesthetic, but in the event the operation becomes longer, excessive amount of local anesthetic may have to be used.

The author prefers a hockey-stick incision extending into the lower quadrant of the abdomen for about 3–4 cm with vertical portion in the proximal thigh, though a longitudinal groin incision is also acceptable. A transverse incision may result in a limited exposure for distal anastomosis to the femoral artery bifurcation or reimplantation of the profunda femoris artery. After subcutaneous tissues are divided, the aneurysm wall is exposed, and attention should then be directed to control the proximal CFA or distal EIA. The origin of the superficial femoral and profunda femoris artery mobilized distally. In most degenerative femoral artery aneurysms, proximal control is obtained close to the origin of the deep epigastric artery and the deep lateral circumflex iliac artery under the inguinal ligament with proximal mobilization aided by a Deaver retractor. In most patients, the deep circumflex iliac vein crossing near the origin of a deep epigastric and lateral deep circumflex iliac artery needs to be ligated and divided to avoid an inadvertent injury resulting in significant blood loss during an exposure.[2] Mobilization of the origin of deep femoral artery can be challenging in patients with large CFA aneurysms. The author prefers intraluminal control with a vascular dilator (Pilling Morrisville, NC) or occlusion catheters after clamping the distal external iliac artery and proximal SFA. The proximal segment of the profunda femoris artery is crossed by a lateral circumflex femoral vein and needs ligation and division in many instances. In very large aneurysms or those presenting with rupture, proximal control is obtained using a short transverse suprainguinal incision.[2] Following therapeutic heparinization by the anesthesia team (ACT between 250 and 300 s), the proximal and distal vascular clamps are applied. Most aneurysms can be completely excised, but for large-sized aneurysms and those surrounded by an inflammatory reaction, partial excision (mostly of the anterior wall) should be performed, as the aneurysm is often adherent to surrounding veins and nerves, risking injury if complete excision of the aneurysm is contemplated.

Excision of large femoral artery aneurysms can result in troublesome postoperative swelling of the extremity due to lymphatic disruption. Type I femoral artery aneurysms, following excision, are reconstructed with proximal CFA-distal CFA interposition graft (Dacron or PTFE) (Figs. 6.2, 6.3, and 6.4).

Type II femoral artery aneurysms are generally repaired with reimplantation of the origin of the deep femoral artery using a 2–3 mm cuff in the opening of the posterolateral aspect of the synthetic graft as a Carrel patch (Fig. 6.5). Occasionally, an interposition graft from the CFA to the profunda femoris is necessary in patients with chronic SFA occlusion with minimal symptoms of arterial occlusion; the interposition graft is anastomosed to the deep femoral artery.

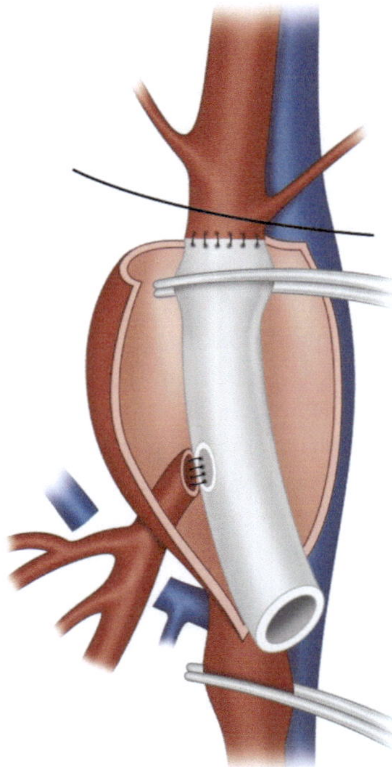

Fig. 6.2 Partial resection of the anterior wall of aneurysm. Vascular clamp applied to the prosthetic graft following completion of proximal end-to-end anastomosis. Vein crossing the deep femoral artery is ligated and divided. The deep femoral artery is being implanted into an opening in the posterolateral wall of the prosthetic graft. Vascular clamp applied to the proximal superficial femoral artery

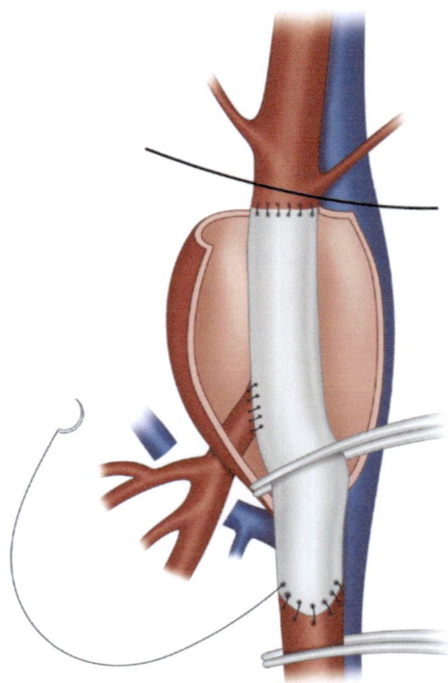

Fig. 6.3 Completed suture line for the deep femoral artery implantation. Completion of distal end-to-end anastomosis of the prosthetic graft to the proximal superficial femoral artery

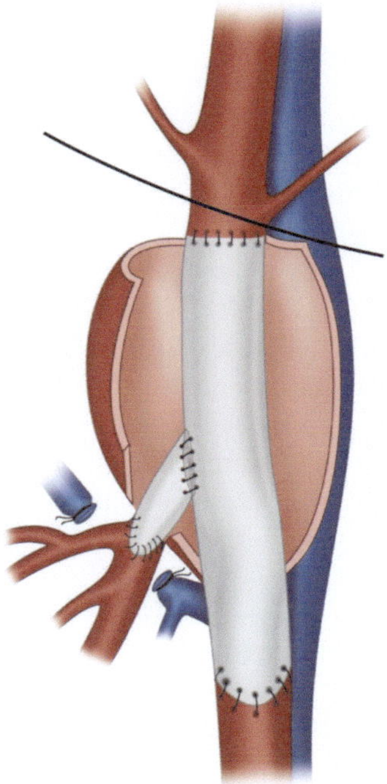

Fig. 6.4 Repair of the right femoral aneurysm with interposition graft. A separate interposition graft from the common femoral artery to superficial femoral artery graft with end-to-end anastomosis and a separate graft to the deep femoral artery

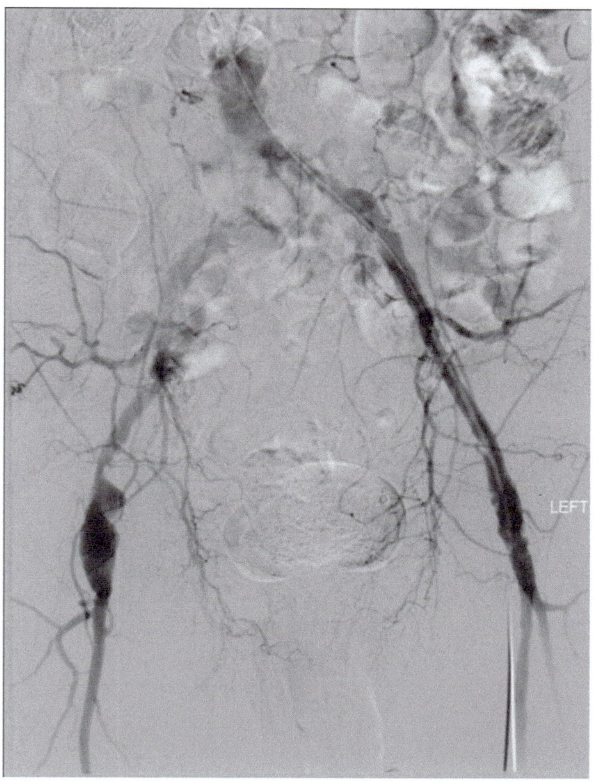

Fig. 6.5 Arteriogram showing the bilateral common femoral artery aneurysm—right larger than the left

Profunda Femoris Artery Aneurysms

Profunda femoris artery aneurysms (PFAAs) are rare and account for only 0.5% of peripheral artery aneurysms and 2.6% of femoral artery aneurysms. It is postulated that several muscles surrounding the PFA and the presence of a rich muscle layer, with paucity of elastic fibers in the profunda femoris artery, prevent aneurysm formation. Most PFAAs are asymptomatic.

Data shows that rupture and acute limb ischemia are uncommon presentations of PFAAs. There is preponderance of men in most reported series of PFAAs, and reported cases suggest that 45%–81% of those patients had other aneurysms. A significant number of patients have shown synchronous aneurysms, with the popliteal artery being the most common site. Aneurysmectomy with a graft interposition from the common femoral artery to the PFA with a synthetic graft (Dacron or PFTE) is the treatment of choice. Ligation of PFA should be avoided; coil embolization may be considered for distal PFA aneurysm in a patient with patent SFA.[3]

Case Example

A 73-year-old man presented to the vascular clinic with symptoms of intermittent claudication in the right calf after walking 50 yards. On examination, he had a pulsatile non-tender mass in the right groin. Duplex imaging of the right groin showed a 3.5-cm-diameter right common femoral artery aneurysm with mural thrombus. Arteriography showed bilateral femoral artery aneurysms with the right larger than the left and a long segment occlusion of the right SFA with reconstitution of the popliteal artery above the knee with three-vessel runoffs (Figs. 6.5 and 6.6). The patient subsequently underwent open repair of the right CFA aneurysm (type I) with interposition of an 8 mm Dacron graft (Gelsoft™ Terumo Tokyo, Japan). A right femoral-popliteal bypass (above the knee) was performed with non-reversed GSV with satisfactory outcome.

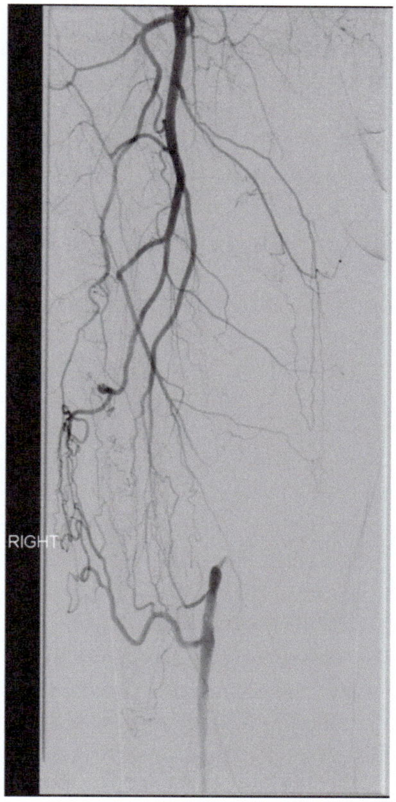

Fig. 6.6 Long-segment right SFA occlusion

Invited Commentary

Introduction

Animesh Rathore, MD, RPVI

This chapter provides a comprehensive overview of a relatively rare but clinically significant condition. The abstract succinctly outlines the key points, including the prevalence, classification, and recommended treatment protocols for these aneurysms. The femoral artery aneurysms are usually asymptomatic and typically diagnosed incidentally on the imaging performed for another indication. However, these may also be found by patients as a pulsatile mass in the groin. Presentation with rupture, occlusion, and distal embolism with acute limb ischemia is rare but has been described.

The chapter effectively classifies femoral artery aneurysms into type I and type II, based on their anatomical location. This distinction is crucial for planning for the appropriate surgical intervention. The epidemiology as well as demographics are well described for the rare condition. The detailed breakdown of aneurysm locations and associated synchronous aneurysms adds depth to the understanding of the condition. Additionally, profunda femoris artery aneurysm is also covered along with the management options. Covered stent-based exclusion is also an option when anatomically feasible, in addition to open surgical repair and coil embolization. Treatment guidelines for the treatment for the symptomatic femoral artery aneurysm as well as a size threshold of 3.5 cm are relevant to the clinical practice. Authors have also included a real-world case scenario, which is commendable. Duplex and CT scan images can potentially add to the diagnostic yield for femoral artery aneurysms for this case.

In addition to the incidence of metachronous aneurysm, arteriomegaly and aneurysmosis are another important consideration. Type I includes aneurysms of the aorta, iliac, and common femoral arteries with arteriomegaly of the superficial femoral and popliteal arteries. Type II includes aneurysms of the common femoral, superficial femoral, and popliteal arteries, with arteriomegaly of the aorta and iliac arteries. Type III includes aneurysms of the aorta, iliac, femoral, and popliteal arteries, with arteriomegaly of the intervening arteries that are not specifically aneurysmal. This is quite relevant in the clinical decision-making as well as can raise suspicion for collagen vascular disorder and might mandate tissue sampling intraoperatively. The use of standard imaging modalities like color-duplex ultrasound, CTA, and MRA is helpful in delineating the anatomical location as well as morphologic differential between true versus pseudoaneurysm. Additional workup is often warranted for anastomotic aneurysm to rule out infectious etiology. Ultimate surgical management is dictated by making sure the proximal and the distal anastomosis includes healthy vessel. Lifelong surveillance is warranted to ensure no late degeneration.

Overall, this chapter on degenerative femoral artery aneurysms is a well-structured and informative piece that effectively covers the essential aspects of the condition. The clear classification, comprehensive data, and practical treatment guidelines are significant strengths.

References

1. Lawrence PF, Harlander-Locke MP, Oderich GS, et al. The current management of isolated degenerative femoral artery aneurysms is too aggressive for their natural history. J Vasc Surg. 2014;59(2):343–9. https://doi.org/10.1016/j.jvs.2013.08.090. PubMed PMID: 24461859.
2. Munie ST, Shepard AD. Open repair of femoral and femoral anastomotic aneurysms. In: Hans SS, editor. Endovascular and open vascular reconstruction: a practical approach. Boca Raton: CRC Press; 2017. p. 263–7.
3. Harbuzariu C, Duncan AA, Bower TC, et al. Profunda femoris artery aneurysms: association with aneurysmal disease and limb ischemia. J Vasc Surg. 2008;47(1):31–4. https://doi.org/10.1016/j.jvs.2007.09.040; discussion 4–5. PubMed PMID: 18178452.

Femoral Artery Pseudoaneurysm Secondary to Femoral Artery Intervention and Penetrating Trauma

7

A pseudoaneurysm (PSA) represents a contained rupture with disruption in the intima, media, and adventitia of the arterial wall. In the lower extremity, it often presents as a pulsatile hematoma. Pseudoaneurysm commonly occurs as a result of a penetrating trauma or following catheterization (coronary and peripheral) for diagnostic purposes, but more commonly it is a result of therapeutic interventions. Pseudoaneurysm results from inadequate sealing of the arterial puncture site with tracking of the blood into tissues surrounding the vessels and the eventual appearance of sac around the puncture site. The surrounding tissues and the contained hematoma form the outer wall of the pseudoaneurysm. Pseudoaneurysm following catheterization is one of the most common vascular complications of coronary and peripheral diagnostic angiography with an incidence rate of 0.05%–2% [1]. In patients undergoing coronary or peripheral intervention, the incidence rate increases to 2%–6% [1]. Femoral pseudoaneurysms are more common following more complex peripheral and coronary interventions.

Spontaneous thrombosis of femoral pseudoaneurysms of less than 3.0 cm was reported in 72 out of 82 patients with a meantime interval of 23 days [1]. It has been reported that spontaneous thrombosis of pseudoaneurysm greater than 1.8 cm with concomitant use of anticoagulation is unlikely to occur. Serial observation of a femoral pseudoaneurysm of less than 2.0 cm without associated severe pain is justified. The more serious complication of PSA is rupture, which is commonly related to its large size (>3 cm), a large hematoma, and the presence of symptoms. In patients under observation of a small-sized aneurysm (<2 cm), any subsequent enlargement or pain is an indication of the need for urgent repair. Although not supported by the literature, it appears anecdotally that the pseudoaneurysms with a wide neck are less likely to spontaneously thrombose as compared to those with a narrow neck.

S. S. Hans, *Contemporary Management of Lower Extremity Aneurysmal Disease*,
https://doi.org/10.1007/978-3-032-00159-7_7

Factors associated with the occurrence of femoral pseudoaneurysm include:

1. High or low puncture sites
2. Large sheath size greater than 7F
3. Age greater than 65 years
4. Peripheral artery disease (PAD)
5. Simultaneous femoral artery and vein puncture
6. Hypertension
7. Patient on hemodialysis
8. Poor post-procedural manual compression
9. Complex intervention

The most important factor for increased incidence of femoral pseudoaneurysm is a high or low puncture site, with puncture not being in the CFA. The complexity of intervention such as coronary stenting/atherectomy, repeat procedure, and intraprocedural use of thrombolytic therapy increases the incidence of PSA. From a systemic review of 34 articles for both diagnostic and peripheral interventions using femoral access, the safety and efficacy were comparable between the use of vascular closure devices (12%) and manual compression (13%) [1]. However, in two studies involving the intention to treat patients undergoing coronary procedures, the incidence of PSA formation was 5.4 times greater when closure devices were used. The availability of prospective data is lacking in order to predict the occurrence of PSA. It has been established that vascular complications are reduced with the use of routine ultrasound for the arterial puncture or fluoroscopy with localization of the femoral head so as to determine the correct position of the common femoral artery and thus enable puncture for entry of the needle on the first attempt.

Diagnosis

The presence of pain or swelling in the groin after femoral artery access is the most common presenting symptom of a femoral artery pseudoaneurysm. Large pseudoaneurysms may cause pain due to compression-associated femoral neuropathy and occasional venous thrombosis. Local necrosis of the skin may occur in large untreated femoral artery pseudoaneurysms. A bruit is often audible over the site of the femoral PSA. In some patients, pain out of proportion to the clinical findings should prompt a femoral artery duplex study. If pain persists after the femoral artery access for intervention (and femoral artery duplex study is negative for pseudoaneurysm), CTA of the pelvis should be obtained. Color Doppler increases the diagnostic accuracy of the ultrasound by identification of the arterial flow in the sac and identification of the neck (Figs. 7.1 and 7.2). When a pulsed Doppler probe is placed within the tract, a "to-and-fro" signal is obtained. In addition to the identification of the loculations and the amount of thrombus within the pseudoaneurysm, the length, depth, and width of the neck connecting the artery to the pseudoaneurysm sac

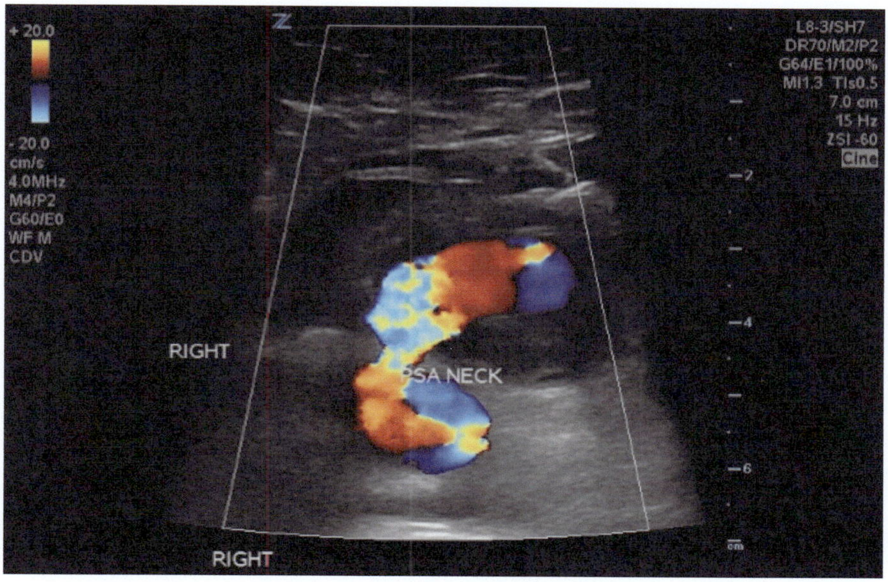

Fig. 7.1 Color duplex imaging of the right common femoral artery showing pseudoaneurysm with a narrow neck

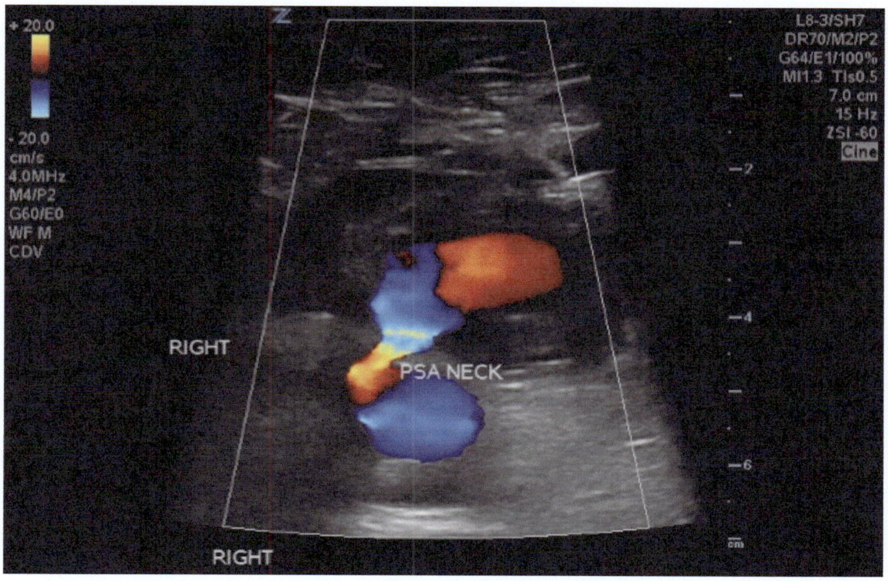

Fig. 7.2 Color duplex imaging of the right common femoral artery showing pseudoaneurysm with a narrow neck

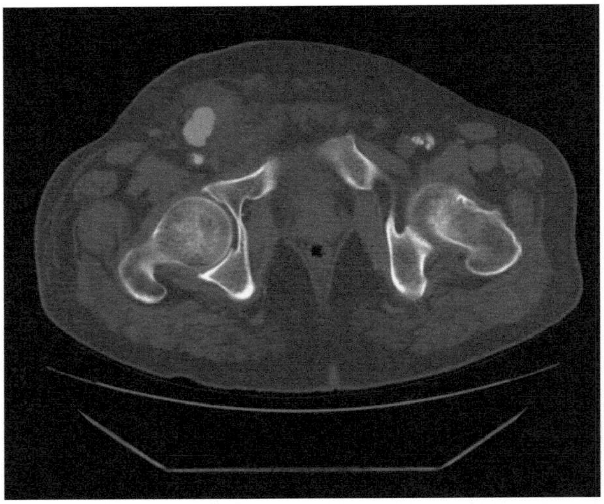

Fig. 7.3 CTA showing large femoral pseudoaneurysm with a short neck

should be identified. The vessel feeding the PSA should be identified in both transverse and longitudinal axes. The flow should also be recorded in the vessel proximal and distal to the PSA. The venous structures should be evaluated for possible deep venous thrombosis. It is also important to increase the depth on the ultrasound machine, so that deep PSAs (>4 cm from the skin) are not missed. The examination should image distal EIA, CFA, and proximal SFA and PFA. The sensitivity of the color-duplex ultrasound for the diagnosis of the PSA is 94% with a specificity of 97%. CTA of the pelvis may be necessary in patients with pseudoaneurysms above the groin and helps in better delineation of the neck (Fig. 7.3).

Management

Prior to the early 1990s, the only treatment available for PSA was surgery. Since then, ultrasound-guided compression, ultrasound-guided thrombin injection, FemoStop compression devices, coil insertion, fibrin adhesives, and balloon occlusion have also been used, but the results of the later procedures are not well documented.

Commonly used modalities for the management of femoral pseudoaneurysms are as follows:

1. Ultrasound-guided compression
2. Ultrasound-guided thrombin injection
3. Surgical repair

Ultrasound-Guided Compression

First introduced in 1991 by Fellmeth et al., the duplex ultrasound is now used to identify the sac and neck (tract) of the PSA, wherein the transducer is positioned, and compression by the transducer is applied to the sac while maintaining arterial flow. Compression is usually applied for cycles of 10 min and can be repeated. Manual compression devices such as FemoStop are easily available; however, the vertical angle created by the device does not allow selective compression of the sac. The lack of nonselective compressions leads to longer compression times, increased patient discomfort, and an inferior success rate with an increased risk of deep vein thrombosis. Higher body mass index (BMI), large size, increased depth of the pseudoaneurysm, and the use of concurrent anticoagulants by patients decrease the success rate of ultrasound-guided compression, but a success rate of 75%–98% has been reported. In patients on anticoagulants, the reported success rate is 30%–73%. Despite initial success, there was recurrence of aneurysm in 10%, with patients requiring subsequent surgical repair.

The main drawback of this method is the amount of time required to achieve the thrombosis, with average reported time of 33 min within a range of 10–120 min. In addition, the procedure is painful and requires concurrent sedation. Rare complications include vasovagal reaction, rupture of PSA, deep vein thrombosis (DVT), and occasionally skin necrosis.

Ultrasound-Guided Thrombin Injection

This is the modality of choice for post-catheterization PSAs. Thrombin injection into the sac of pseudoaneurysm near its neck results in conversion of fibrinogen to fibrin, resulting in instantaneous formation of a fibrin clot even among patients on anticoagulants. A success rate of 91%–100% has been reported in many studies [2].

Bovine thrombin is available in a commercial kit, and it is generally reconstituted in NS to a concentration of 1000 units per mL.

Technique After obtaining informed consent, the groin is prepped with ChloraPrep, and time-out is called, and distal pulses (DP/PT) are palpated. In patients with poor or absent distal pulses, preprocedure arterial Doppler study including ABIs should be obtained. The injection site is prepared in a sterile fashion, and 1%–2% lidocaine is infiltrated into the skin and subcutaneous tissues. A three-way stopcock technique is used with NS placed into a 5 mL syringe via 22-guage needle (Fig. 7.4). In most instances, a 1.5 inch 22 gauge needle is used. In patients with deeper PSA (>3.75 cm from the skin), a 21 gauge by 9 cm needle EchoTip (Cook Inc., Bloomington, IN) that can be visualized by ultrasound is preferred. With the thrombin stopcock turned off and the saline stopcock in place, the needle is advanced under the guidance of the ultrasound. The needle and the transducer are positioned in parallel to the puncture of the sac of the pseudoaneurysm and should be kept away from the neck (tract) of the PSA [2]. The B-mode imaging is better able to visualize the needle tip [2].

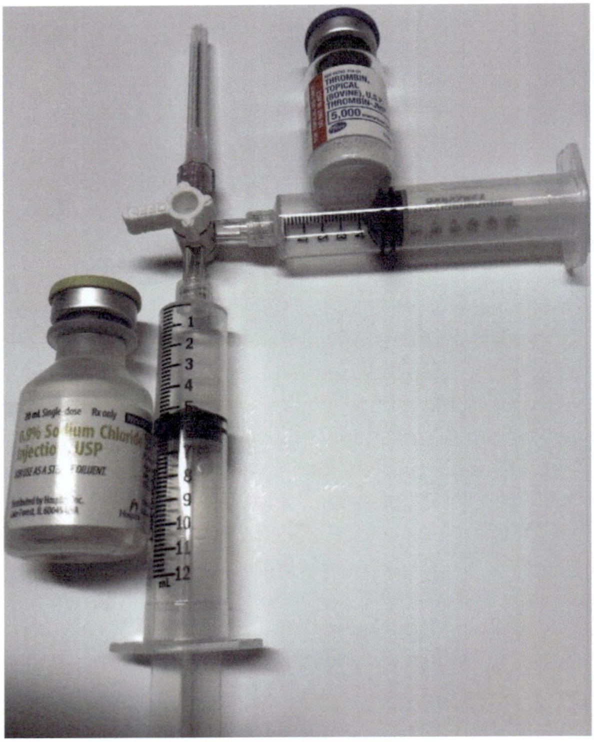

Fig. 7.4 Preparation of thrombin injection into pseudoaneurysm

The confirmation of the proper needle placement is done with aspiration of the arterial blood and the small amount of injection of saline to produce color flash in the aneurysm sac. Once the needle tip is in the satisfactory position, the stopcock in the thrombin is turned "on," and the saline stopcock is turned off. Aliquots (0.2 mL) are injected into the sac and visualized into color Doppler until no flow is detected, all of which takes place in a few seconds. A follow-up ultrasound is performed the following day. The direct injection into the tract neck of the pseudoaneurysm is avoided as it may result in thrombosis of the artery. In most patients, 0.2–0.4 mL of thrombin is required. Distal pulses are palpated, and if absent preprocedure, Doppler flow in DP/PT is evaluated. The recurrence rate of 0%–0.9% has been reported in the follow-up imaging obtained the next day. Recurrence can be treated with a second or even third injection. The most serious complications include deep vein thrombosis of the native artery. The author tends to avoid thrombin injection in pseudoaneurysm with a wide short neck. Allergic and anaphylactic reactions have been reported in patients previously exposed to bovine thrombin. Thrombin injection should be avoided in patient with mycotic pseudoaneurysm.

Surgical repair Patients with very large pseudoaneurysm with or without skin necrosis, compression of surrounding structures (nerve or vein), or severe pain should undergo surgical repair. The author also prefers surgical repair in patient with a wide (>3–4 mm) short neck (tract) or in instances when the neck is not well visualized in the axis of the ultrasound profile.

Technique A hockey-stick incision is made in the groin over the site of the pulsatile mass. Incision should extend at least 5 cm proximal to the puncture site in the skin, and subcutaneous tissues are incised. In most instances, a large hematoma is seen.

A large self-retaining retractor such as a Weitlaner or Beckman-Adson retractor in obese patients (Pilling Surgical, Morrisville, NC) is applied. In many patients, the active bleeding from the puncture site will start during retraction. A proximal and distal compression is applied with a Kittner sponge to the artery at the site of the bleeding, and one horizontal mattress suture of "5.0" cardiovascular polypropylene (Ethicon, Raritan, NJ) is applied. In patients with larger than 2 mm opening in the artery, an additional suture is often necessary. The hematoma is evacuated manually, and in patients with large pseudoaneurysms, suction drainage with Jackson-Pratt drain is recommended. There is often persistent serosanguinous drainage for at least 3–4 days after repair. Wound complications are not uncommon following open repair of femoral PSA.

Case Example

A 64-year-old man had significant bruising and painful swelling of the right groin following cardiac catheterization using right femoral approach and a Perclose device for closure. A femoral duplex study showed a pseudoaneurysm, but a CTA was needed to see an aneurysm that was 3.2–3.5 cm in diameter. The neck was short and curbing, which made it more challenging to perform thrombin injections; therefore, an open repair was necessary.

A hockey-stick-shaped incision was made in the right groin, and subcutaneous tissues were incised. The pseudoaneurysm was exposed; a large amount of thrombosis was removed from the aneurysm, and it had a pulsatile flow from the opening in the femoral artery. A Kittner sponge was placed proximally and distally to provide manual pressure and visualize the opening in the common femoral artery. A 5–0 cardiovascular Prolene horizontal mattress suture was used.

Invited Commentary

NavYash Gupta, MD, FACS

As vascular surgeons, we are frequently asked to see patients in consultation in the hospital and on occasion in the outpatient setting for femoral artery pseudoaneurysms following peripheral and coronary interventions. On occasion, we see these patients following inadvertent femoral artery puncture in the process of femoral venous access.

The author describes quite well the numerous factors that can predispose to the development of these pseudoaneurysms as well as the various treatment modalities. Routine use of ultrasound guidance for femoral artery access can help reduce the incidence of high or low punctures, both of which increase the incidence of pseudoaneurysm development.

Ultrasound-guided thrombin injection has facilitated the treatment of the majority of these pseudoaneurysms with a safe and effective modality. In patients with relatively wide and/or short necks, temporary balloon occlusion of the femoral artery during thrombin injection can still enable this treatment method. CT angiography may allow for better visualization of the anatomy in patients where the anatomy and neck are poorly imaged on ultrasonography. Open repair remains a durable method of treatment, albeit associated with greater morbidity and potential wound complications.

References

1. Webber GW, Jang J, Gustavson S, Olin JW. Contemporary management of postcatheterization pseudoaneurysms. Circulation. 2007;115(20):2666–74. https://doi.org/10.1161/circulationaha.106.681973. PubMed PMID: 17515479.
2. Khoury M, Rebecca A, Greene K, et al. Duplex scanning-guided thrombin injection for the treatment of iatrogenic pseudoaneurysms. J Vasc Surg. 2002;35(3):517–21. https://doi.org/10.1067/mva.2002.120029. PubMed PMID: 11877701.

Femoral Artery Anastomotic Aneurysms

8

Femoral artery anastomotic aneurysms (FAAs) often occur as a late complication after aortofemoral reconstruction with a prosthetic graft for occlusive or aneurysmal disease of the aortoiliac arterial segment. The reported incidence varies from 2 to 29%, depending on the screening method for its detection and duration of follow-up [1]. The low incidence of 2% is probably a reflection of incomplete follow-up. The reported incidence of FAAs after 15 years of aortofemoral reconstruction is approximately 25% [1]. FAAs commonly occur 5 years following primary aortofemoral reconstruction. The exact cause for the development of FAAs is not known, but contributing factors include type of suture material, anastomotic stress resulting from compliance mismatch, repeated hip flexion, multiple reconstructions, trauma, perioperative anticoagulation, wound healing complications—such as lymphorrhea or hematoma—and excessive tension at the anastomosis. In the 1960s, the silk suture was used for arterial anastomosis with eventual fraying of the suture that resulted in high incidence of FAAs. Since the widespread use of polypropylene suture in the mid-1970s, the deterioration of the suture material is not a significant contributing factor in the development of FAAs [1]. The degeneration of the arterial wall is considered an important factor in causing FAA; we have not encountered infection as the cause of most FAAs. However, reports of postoperative surgical site infection in the groin with positive bacteriological cultures and lymph have been reported in patients diagnosed with late FAAs. Seabrook et al. reported coagulase-negative staphylococcal infection in 60% of femoral anastomotic aneurysms [2].

Diagnosis Diagnosis can be suspected in patients presenting with a pulsatile mass in the groin area at the site incision. Color-duplex ultrasound confirms the diagnosis with determination of the exact size of the aneurysm and anatomy of the inflow and outflow of vessels (Figs. 8.1 and 8.2). CT angiography of the entire graft should be obtained to detect proximal aortic abdominal aneurysm (AA) and to rule out the remote possibility of infection (gas bubbles or fluid) around the graft. CT angiography helps in planning operative repair (Fig. 8.3).

S. S. Hans, *Contemporary Management of Lower Extremity Aneurysmal Disease*,
https://doi.org/10.1007/978-3-032-00159-7_8

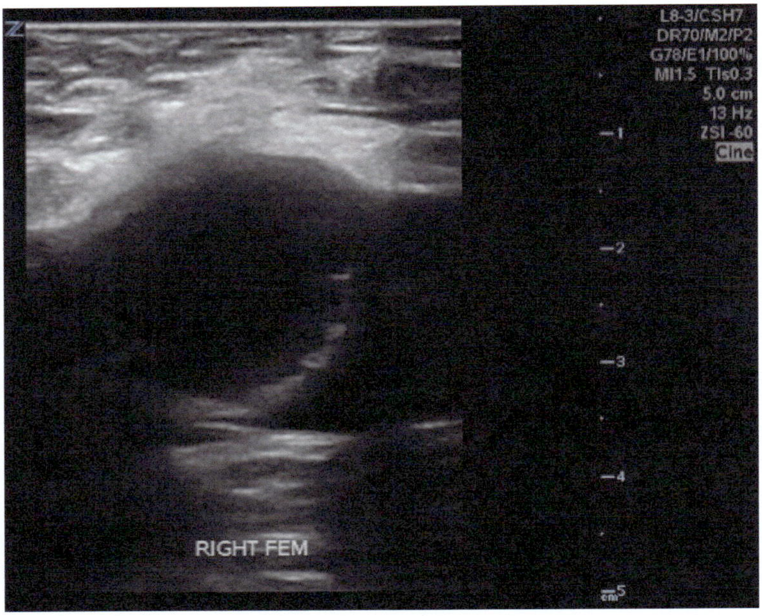

Fig. 8.1 Duplex ultrasound demonstrating femoral anastomotic aneurysm

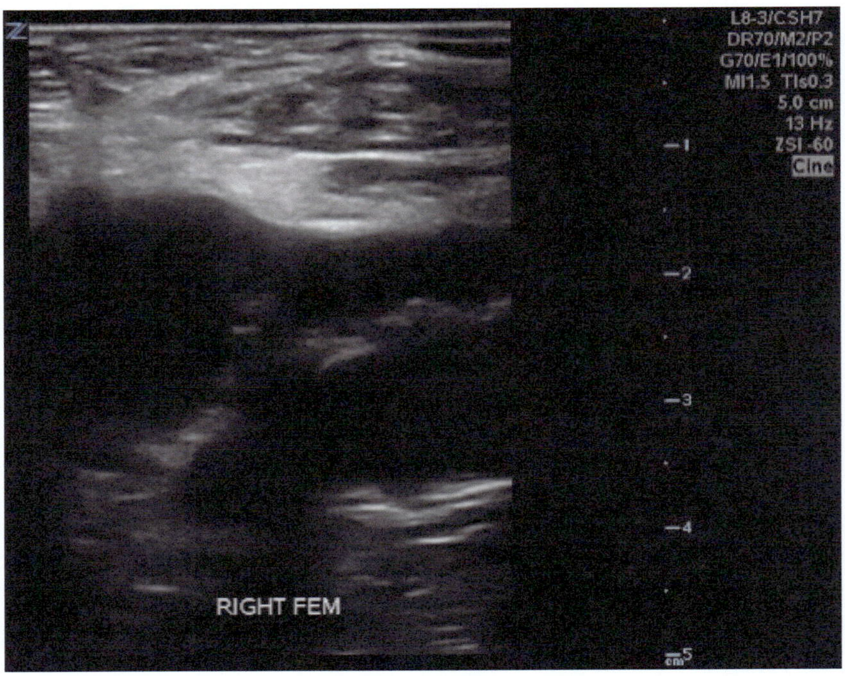

Fig. 8.2 Duplex ultrasound demonstrating femoral anastomotic aneurysm

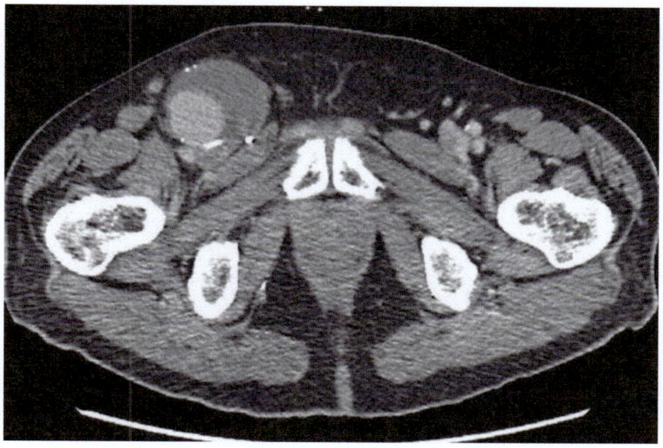

Fig. 8.3 CTA showing right femoral anastomotic aneurysm

Management Femoral AAs smaller than 2.5 cm can be safely observed with clinical exam and surveillance color-duplex ultrasound imaging. Femoral AAs larger than 2.5 cm in transverse/AP diameter should undergo repair, except in patients with extremely poor medical condition.

Open repair The groin (inguinal) scar from the aortofemoral reconstruction is extended proximally and distally. The proximal incision is extended horizontally, and its distal portion is extended vertically so that the incision is in a hockey-stick configuration. The subcutaneous tissues are incised using electrocautery or with a scalpel exposing the outer wall of the aneurysm. The proximal exposure under the inguinal ligament is performed by proximal retraction using a "baby" Deaver retractor (Integra LifeSciences Princeton, NJ). The well-incorporated limb of the aortofemoral graft is exposed (Fig. 8.4). The outer sheath (fibrous) of the graft is incised to expose the underlying synthetic graft. The graft is usually well incorporated. In most patients, the CFA proximal to the anastomosis is either of a small caliber or even occluded. Dissecting the proximal CFA and external iliac artery junction posterior to the graft can be challenging, and injury to the artery may result in troublesome bleeding. The author recommends intraluminal control after the aneurysm is opened and proximal and distal control has been obtained. The dense scar tissue around the outer wall of the anastomosis aneurysm necessitates a sharp dissection with a 15 blade scalpel at an angle. The medial wall of the aneurysm is often adherent to the common femoral vein, and it is not necessary to dissect it from the vein to reduce the chance of troublesome bleeding. The attention is then directed to obtaining distal control. Proximal SFA is exposed, and silastic vessel loop is passed. The exposure of the deep femoral artery may be cumbersome in patients with large femoral anastomotic aneurysms, and dissection is done to expose the vein crossing the deep femoral artery (lateral circumflex femoral vein); intraluminal control with a number 5 or 6 Garrett arterial dilator (Integra LifeSciences, Princeton, NJ) is preferable. Systemic heparin (100 units/kg) is administered by the anesthesia team. The aneurysm is opened after vascular clamps are applied to the graft limb, SFA, and

Fig. 8.4 Femoral anastomotic aneurysm

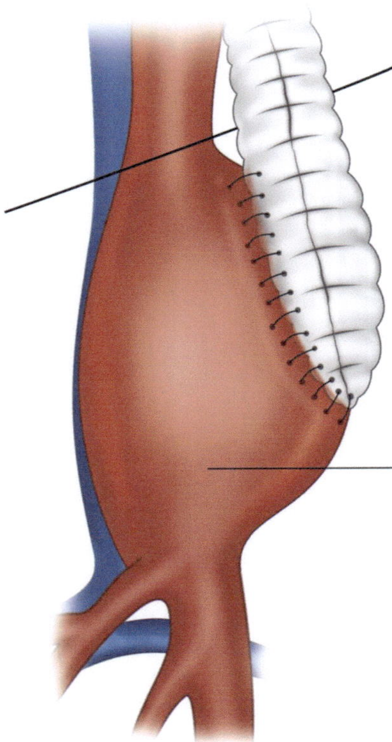

deep femoral artery. In situations where exposure of deep femoral artery is not feasible due to large size of the anastomotic aneurysm, intraluminal control with a Garrett dilator or a No. 5 Fogarty balloon catheter should be considered (Fig. 8.5).

After opening the anterior wall of the aneurysm, thrombus is removed, and any retrograde bleeding such as from native proximal common femoral artery is controlled by number 5 or 6 Garrett dilator (Fig. 8.6), which is also carefully controlled. The suture line of the previously placed femoral anastomosis of the aortofemoral graft is dissected, and the graft is then circumferentially removed from the host artery (CFA and proximal SFA). We take routine cultures from the wall of the synthetic graft and the lumen (thrombus) of the contents of the aneurysm. After excision of the aneurysm, an 8-mm-diameter interposition graft (Dacron or PTFE) is selected, and proximal anastomosis is performed end-to-end with the graft limb of the aortofemoral graft (index operator) using 4′0″ CV polypropylene suture (Ethicon, Rariton, NJ) and distal anastomosis at the distal CFA in an end-to-end manner with a 5″0″ CV polypropylene suture in an oblique manner incorporating the origin of the SFA and DFA at the anastomosis. The posterior wall of distal CFA may not have to be completely transected and can be used as a double layer and sutured to obliquely divided synthetic graft using 4′0″–5′0″ CV polypropylene suture depending upon the quality of the arterial wall.

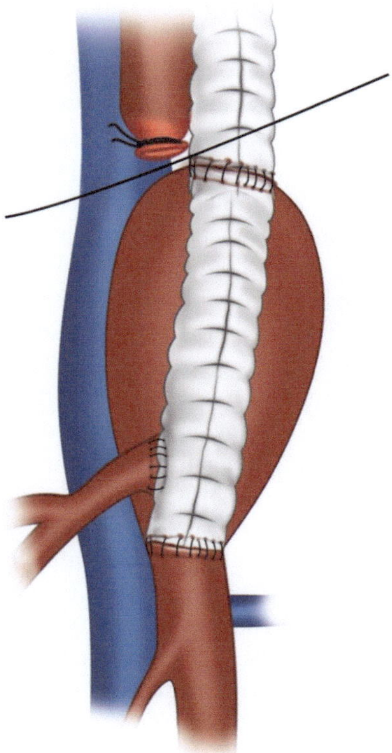

Fig. 8.5 Repair of femoral anastomotic aneurysm with interposition graft and reimplantation of the deep femoral artery into newly interposed prosthetic graft

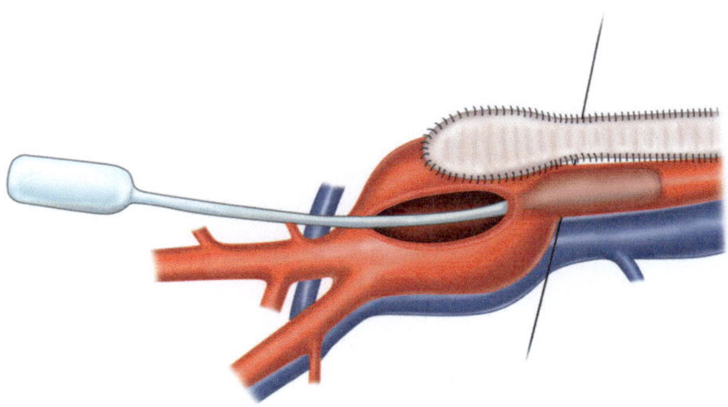

Fig. 8.6 Control of native proximal common femoral artery with appropriately sized arterial dilator

In some instances, deep femoral artery with a cuff of the arterial wall is sutured to an opening in the posterolateral wall of the interposition graft as a carrel patch or a separate graft (usually 6 mm Dacron/PTFE) that is anastomosed to the deep femoral artery from an opening in the interposition graft as described in the Chap. 9 on femoral artery aneurysm (Fig. 9.7). The wound is closed in layers with PICO dressing negative wound pressure therapy (Smith & Nephew Plc., Watford, England).

Postoperative Complications

1. Hemorrhage (postoperative bleeding) secondary to the large area of dissection with diffuse oozing in the subcutaneous tissue and formation of a hematoma that is usually self-contained: suture line bleeding is extremely uncommon.
2. Lymphatic leaks and lymphoceles are common and can be avoided by careful ligation of the lymphatics during the exposure. Despite a careful technique, the lymphatic fistulas occur at an incidence of approximately 1.1% in patients undergoing lower extremity vascular reconstruction. This is mostly due to lymph leak from prominent lymphatic channels. The important contributing factors to the formation of lymphocele and lymphatic fistula include failure to ligate or electrocoagulate lymphatics, inadequate closure of all tissue layers, and patients with associated diabetes mellitus. The diagnosis of lymphatic fistula is made by the persistent leakage of clear yellowish fluid. Early diagnosis and management are important to prevent future complications. Lymphoscintigraphy is rarely needed except when the lymphatic leakage occurs several months after arterial reconstruction. A CT scan should be obtained to exclude a vascular graft infection. Patient presenting with lymphocele a few weeks later after reconstruction should be evaluated by CT scan and taken to the operating room for drainage of the lymphocele, ligation of leaking lymphatics, and careful closure in the layers without any dead space. Initially, conservative management with antibiotics, local wound management, bed rest, and elevation are required to decrease the amount of lymph flow.
3. Infection is a rare complication of anastomotic aneurysm repair and may present as cellulitis of the overlying skin, which often responds to antibiotics used for skin microorganisms. Deeper infection should be clinically evaluated, and imaging studies should be performed to prevent secondary hemorrhage. There is also a reported higher incidence of recurrent anastomotic aneurysms in patients with postoperative infection. Most deep surgical site infections (SSI) will need evaluation by CT scan, functional radionuclide imaging (indium-labelled leukocytes or 99m Tc-hexametazine-labelled leukocytes), which can confirm the presence of a clinically suspected graft infection in patients with equivocal signs of graft infection.

Vacuum-assisted closure (VAC) therapy is useful for the management of lymphocutaneous fistula in patients undergoing LE bypass. Following repair of FAA, lymphocutaneous fistula should be managed by operative exploration after injection of isosulfan blue dye into the first and third interdigital spaces of the foot, and sequential compression pump is placed over the affected leg to increase venous and lymphatic drainage. During operative exploration, leakage of blue dye aids in the identification of lymphatic injury. The leaky lymphatic is sutured with nonabsorbable sutures, and the wound is closed in layers.

Lymphocele Lymphocele is a localized collection of lymph that develops between two planes of tissues and is not reabsorbed. Compared to seroma, a lymphocele has a well-localized connection with the lymphatic channels. Lymphoscintigraphy can readily diagnose a lymphocele. Large lymphoceles cause local discomfort and pain with mild swelling of the LE [3].

Seroma and SSI infection should be considered differential in diagnosis. The presence of a soft, fluid-filled cyst with intermittent drainage of clear lymph from the fistula confirms the diagnosis of lymphocele. Ultrasonography can distinguish a solid dense hematoma from a cystic lymphocele [3]. CT scan is helpful in excluding graft infection or identifying a retroperitoneal lymphocele extending to the groin [3]. Small lymphocele may get absorbed spontaneously, but a large lymphocele and those near the synthetic graft should undergo surgical intervention to decrease the potential of graft infection [2].

Invited Commentary

Dipankar Mukherjee, MD, FACS, DFSVS

The manuscript detailing operative repair of a common problem following aorta to bilateral common femoral artery bypass (AFB), which had been the standard repair for advanced occlusive disease of the distal aorta and iliac arteries, was extremely informative and illustrative. Despite the advances of endovascular therapy and certainly following failed endovascular therapy, AFB remains the treatment of choice for many patients.

Dr. Hans reminds us that "femoral artery anastomotic aneurysms" are a significant problem with an incidence of 25% after 15 years of follow-up of patients who have undergone AFB repair.

He has carefully described surgical control of the common femoral artery (CFA), profunda femoris artery (PFA), and the superficial femoral artery (SFA) in a scarred groin, which can indeed be challenging. He states explicitly that there is no need for circumferential control of the CFA and PFA risking major bleeding.

Vascular surgery trainees and young attending surgeons will benefit from the intraoperative details of using a vascular dilator or balloon occlusion to prevent retrograde bleeding from the proximal CFA or PFA.

He reminds us of the value of careful follow-up of all patients and the value of CTA to evaluate the proximal anastomosis of the AFB for a proximal anastomotic aneurysm as well.

In this era of endovascular revolution of the management of vascular disease, it was refreshing to read a lucid description of open repair of "femoral artery anastomotic aneurysms."

References

1. Mulder EJ, van Bockel JH, Maas J, et al. Morbidity and mortality of reconstructive surgery of noninfected false aneurysms detected long after aortic prosthetic reconstruction. Arch Surg. 1998;133(1):45–9. https://doi.org/10.1001/archsurg.133.1.45. PubMed PMID: 9438758.
2. Seabrook GR, Schmitt DD, Bandyk DF, et al. Anastomotic femoral pseudoaneurysm: an investigation of occult infection as an etiologic factor. J Vasc Surg. 1990;11(5):629–34. https://doi.org/10.1067/mva.1990.19708. PubMed PMID: 2139897.
3. Davis F, Henke P. Complications of femoropopliteal and infrapopliteal artery bypass. In: Hans SS, editor. Vascular and endovascular complications – a practical approach. Boca Raton: CRC Press; 2021. p. 220–32.

Complex Femoral Anastomotic Aneurysms

9

Diagnosis and repair of most femoral anastomotic aneurysms (FAAs) are straightforward, and its repair is associated with a low mortality and morbidity rate. However, there are certain categories of FAAs, with complex presentations that may necessitate technically challenging arterial reconstruction.

The categories of patient with complex FAAs include:

A. Large size >5 cm
B. Recurrent
C. Rupture (leaking)
D. Acute thrombosis
E. Those requiring simultaneous lower extremity arterial reconstruction for associated severe lower extremity ischemia

A. *Large femoral anastomotic aneurysm (FAA)*—Patients with large femoral AAs (greater than 5 cm in diameter) often present with pain and associated symptoms of femoral cutaneous neuropathy due to compression of the femoral nerve branches and occasional swelling of the lower extremity due to extrinsic compression of the femoral vein [1–4]. Large-sized femoral AAs, if untreated, can rupture and result in severe pain and occasional hypotension. Rupture may not be considered in differential diagnosis because hypotension is often not as profound as compared to a rupture of the AAA or iliac artery aneurysm. For very large FAAs, a suprainguinal incision enables the dissection to be carried out in a retroperitoneal plane for exposure of the limb of the aortofemoral graft in order to obtain proximal control. Control of the profunda femoris artery can be challenging, and the author prefers intraluminal control with Garrett's arterial dilator or a balloon catheter occlusion after obtaining proximal control of the femoral limb of the graft and distal control of the proximal superficial femoral artery (SFA). In most instances, native proximal common femoral artery (CFA) needs to be ligated.

S. S. Hans, *Contemporary Management of Lower Extremity Aneurysmal Disease*,
https://doi.org/10.1007/978-3-032-00159-7_9

B. *Recurrent femoral anastomotic aneurysms*—Repair of recurrent femoral AAs can be challenging like most repeat arterial reconstructions. The factors associated with recurrence include local wound complications after initial aortofemoral graft reconstruction or the development of femoral AA within 4.5 years or after aortofemoral grafting. Recurrent FAAs are more common in women. In patients with significant comorbidities, it is prudent to observe recurrent femoral anastomotic aneurysms of less than 3.0 cm in transverse/AP diameter.

   In some patients with large recurrent femoral AAs, proximal control should be obtained by exposing the femoral limb of the aortofemoral graft via a suprainguinal incision.
C. *Rupture*—Most patients with a contained rupture have a hematoma in the groin and proximal thigh, for which emergent repair is required. Proximal control is obtained using a suprainguinal incision with retroperitoneal (RP) exposure. The remaining procedure is carried out as for an uncomplicated aneurysm following adequate fluid resuscitation by the anesthesia team.
D. *Thrombosis*—Thrombosis of the femoral AA is uncommon but often requires urgent repair in patients presenting with acute ischemia of the lower extremity (LE).
E. *Patients requiring simultaneous lower extremity arterial reconstruction*—Some patients with prior aortofemoral grafting presenting femoral AA with associated severe lower extremity arterial occlusive disease will require open repair of anastomotic aneurysm and simultaneous infrainguinal bypass. The origin of the great saphenous vein is anastomosed to the distal portion of the femoral interposition graft as a composite graft is anastomosed to the proximal portion of SFA. Occasionally, patient may present femoral AA in the presence of a crossover femoral-femoral graft. After repairing the femoral AA, the crossover femoral-femoral graft is anastomosed to the femoral interposition graft and may require an additional short interposition graft as the femoral-femoral graft may not reach the new interposition graft following repair of the anastomotic aneurysm.

Repair of large and recurrent FAAs carries similar morbidity and mortality rates to that of the repair of primary FAAs. Patients presenting with thrombosis and rupture have a higher morbidity and mortality rate than repair of primary FAA.

Case Example 1

A 62-year-old woman presented to her primary care physician with a large pulsatile mass in the left groin and a smaller mass in the right groin. She had a prior aortobifemoral graft followed by a redo aortobifemoral graft performed many years previously. Duplex ultrasound showed 5.5 cm left femoral anastomotic aneurysm and 3.5 cm right femoral anastomotic aneurysm, and a CTA of the abdomen and pelvis confirmed these findings (Fig. 9.1). The patient underwent open repair in December 2020 using a left suprainguinal transverse incision. Proximal control was obtained

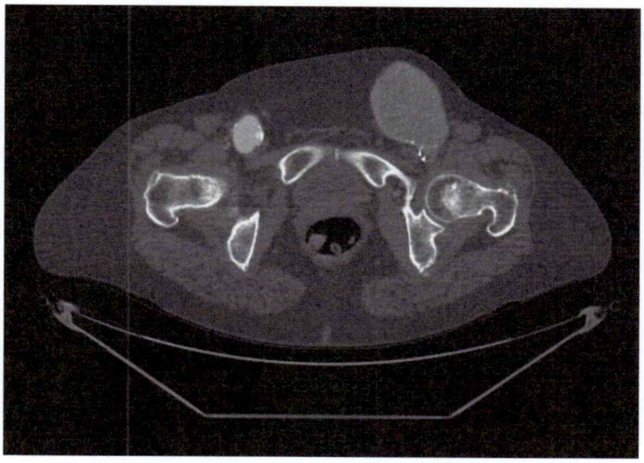

Fig. 9.1 CTA pelvis showing a large femoral anastomotic aneurysm and a smaller right femoral anastomotic aneurysm

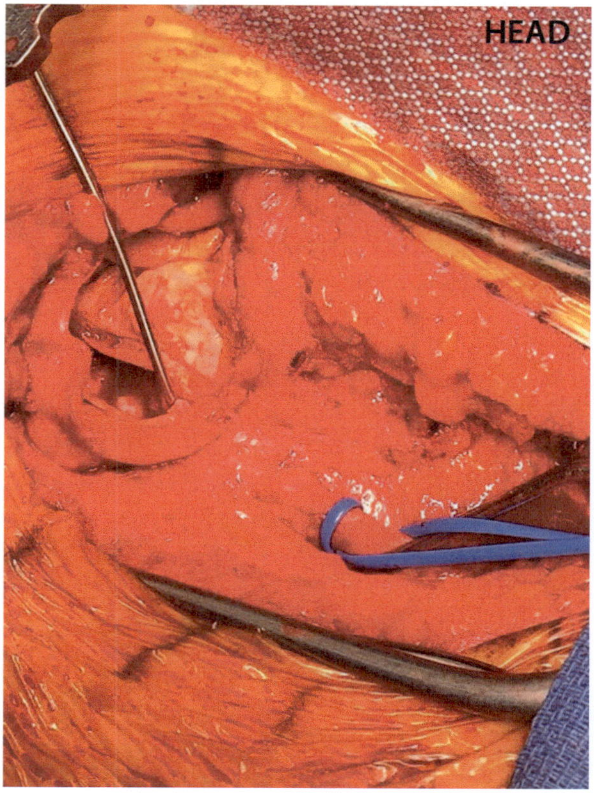

Fig. 9.2 Proximal superficial femoral artery controlled with a silastic loop

of the left limb of the aortofemoral graft, and large left femoral anastomotic aneurysm was exposed. Proximal superficial femoral artery (SFA) was controlled with silastic vessel loop and intraluminal control of the profunda femoris artery with a No. 5 Garrett arterial dilator after an opening of the large aneurysm (Fig. 9.2) was obtained. An interposition 8 mm Dacron graft was anastomosed proximally to the left limb of the aortobifemoral graft end-to-end, and distal anastomosis was also

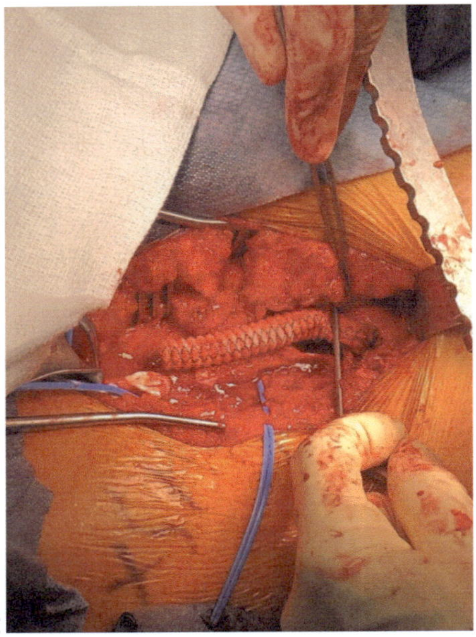

Fig. 9.3 Interposition Dacron graft from the proximal CFA to proximal SFA

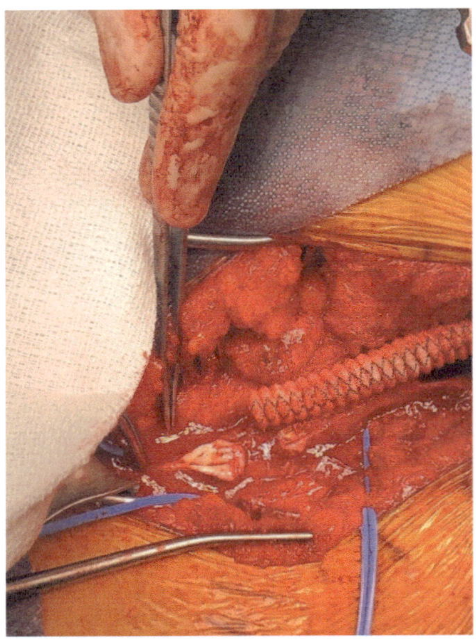

Fig. 9.4 Showing spatulated profunda femoris artery with interposition Dacron graft

performed end-to-end to the proximal SFA (Fig. 9.3). The deep profunda femoris artery was anastomosed with a Carrel patch to an opening in the posterolateral aspect of the interposition graft (Figs. 9.4, 9.5, and 9.6). Follow-up duplex imaging showed elevated peak systolic velocity in the proximal left SFA. Patient underwent

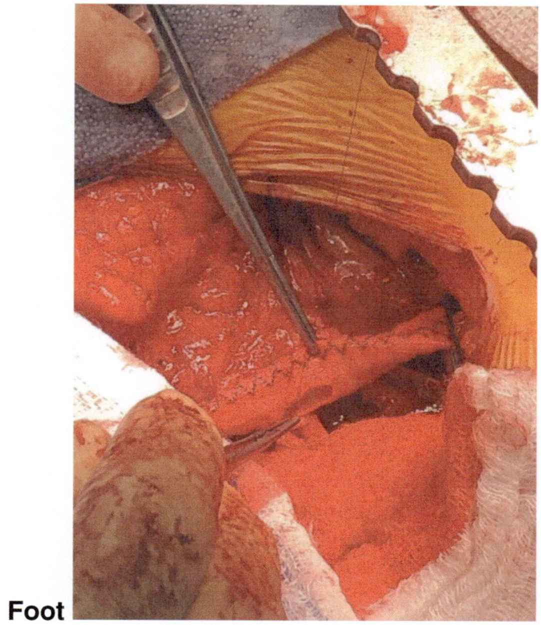

Fig. 9.5 Opening made in interposition Dacron graft

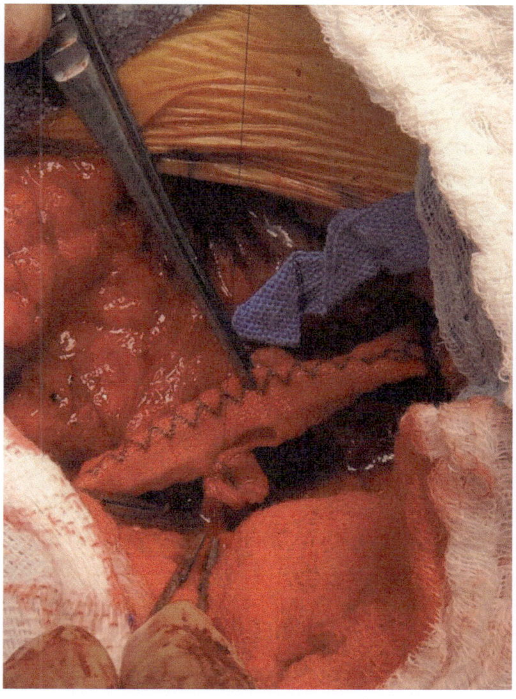

Fig. 9.6 Profunda femoris after being anastomosed to the posterolateral opening in the interposition graft

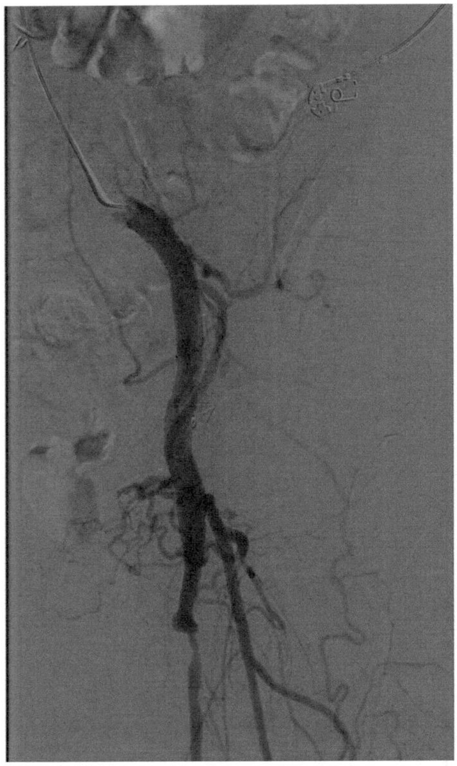

Fig. 9.7 Follow-up arteriogram of the left lower extremity 3 years later showing patient's interposition graft and implanted deep femoral artery with moderate stenosis in the proximal superficial femoral artery

repair of the contralateral femoral anastomotic aneurysm in 2021. The patient underwent left SFA angioplasty using left brachial access in October 2023. Anastomosis of the deep femoral artery into interposition graft (end-to-side) was widely patent (Fig. 9.7).

Case Example 2

A 59-year-old man with pain in the right groin and ecchymosis of 48 h duration came to the emergency room (ER) (Fig. 9.8). The patient had undergone aortobifemoral graft 4 years prior for an aortoiliac occlusive disease. The initial impression in the ER suggested an incarcerated right groin hernia. A contrast-enhanced CT scan of the abdomen and pelvis showed a leaking right femoral anastomotic aneurysm (Fig. 9.9). The patient underwent emergency repair with interposition of an 8 mm Dacron graft from the right limb of the aortobifemoral graft to the deep femoral artery because SFA was chronically occluded. The patient was last seen in the clinic in July 2023 with patent aortobifemoral graft and was asymptomatic without recurrence of femoral anastomotic aneurysm.

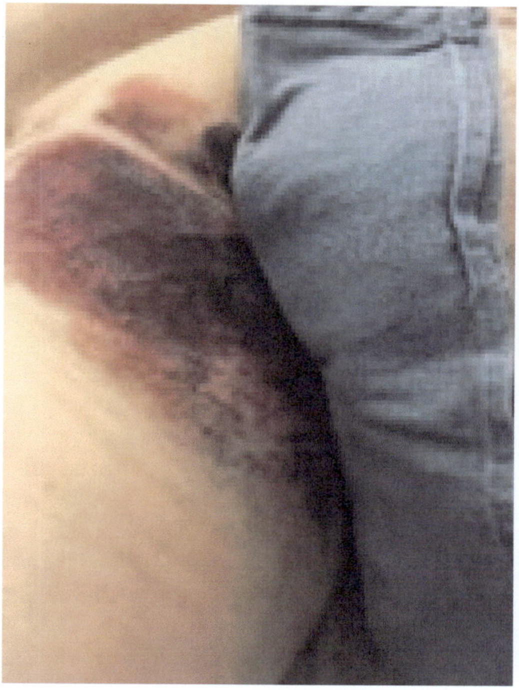

Fig. 9.8 Groin ecchymosis from leaking femoral AA

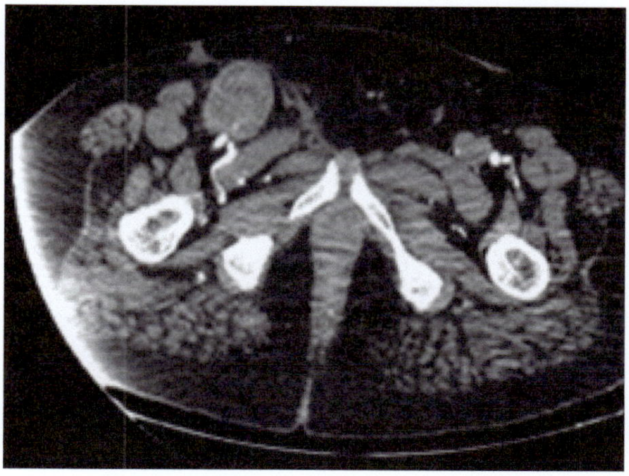

Fig. 9.9 CTA pelvis showing leaking femoral anastomotic aneurysm

Invited Commentary

Dipankar Mukherjee, MD, FACS, DFSVS

In this chapter, Dr. Hans has detailed open surgical management of large and complex femoral artery anastomotic aneurysms.

While embracing the age-old truths of vascular reconstruction of proximal and distal control, he instructs us to "tame the tiger" by retroperitoneal exposure and control of the limb of the AFB graft before exposing the CFA, PFA, and proximal SFA.

Heeding this advice is likely to lead to safe conduct of the operation and could prevent life-threatening hemorrhage.

Evaluation of the outflow vessels is just as important as he has shown in the two case examples discussed in the chapter. In one, the PFA alone was patent, and direct end-to-end anastomosis was performed to this vessel, while in the other, both the SFA and PFA were patent. Reconstruction was by end-to-end anastomosis to the SFA, and the PFA was reimplanted into the lateral aspect of the interposition graft.

This chapter dovetails perfectly with the previous Chap. 8. The pearls offered in the previous chapter should be included with the measures recommended in this chapter to guide the surgeon in the safe and efficient management of "femoral artery anastomotic aneurysms."

References

1. Ylönen K, Biancari F, Leo E, et al. Predictors of development of anastomotic femoral pseudoaneurysms after aortobifemoral reconstruction for abdominal aortic aneurysm. Am J Surg. 2004;187(1):83–7. https://doi.org/10.1016/j.amjsurg.2002.09.001. PubMed PMID: 14706592.
2. Mulder EJ, van Bockel JH, Maas J, et al. Morbidity and mortality of reconstructive surgery of noninfected false aneurysms detected long after aortic prosthetic reconstruction. Arch Surg. 1998;133(1):45–9. https://doi.org/10.1001/archsurg.133.1.45. PubMed PMID: 9438758.
3. Levi N, Schroeder TV. True and anastomotic femoral artery aneurysms: is the risk of rupture and thrombosis related to the size of the aneurysms? Eur J Vasc Endovasc Surg. 1999;18(2):111–3. https://doi.org/10.1053/ejvs.1999.0842. PubMed PMID: 10426967.
4. Seabrook GR, Schmitt DD, Bandyk DF, et al. Anastomotic femoral pseudoaneurysm: an investigation of occult infection as an etiologic factor. J Vasc Surg. 1990;11(5):629–34. https://doi.org/10.1067/mva.1990.19708. PubMed PMID: 2139897.

Mycotic Femoral Artery Aneurysms 10

The term mycotic aneurysm was first used by William Osler in 1885, which alludes to localized irreversible dilation of an artery due to vessel wall destruction by infection. This may occur in a proximal normal artery or occasionally due to secondary infection involving a preexisting aneurysm, the latter case being rare.

The common causes include:

1. Bacteremia from a distant source with bacterial colonization in the wall of the femoral artery
2. Bacterial endocarditis causing septic emboli in the arterial tree
3. Intravenous drug abuse
4. Synthetic graft infection

Mycotic Femoral Artery Pseudoaneurysm due to Intravenous Drug Abuse

Infected mycotic femoral artery pseudoaneurysm is a well-known complication in patients with parenteral drug abuse. It is due to an accidental or a deliberate intra-arterial drug infection (Fig. 10.1). The pathogenesis of infected femoral artery pseudoaneurysm most often consists of the introduction of infected material by a non-sterile needle combined with arterial trauma; some access to peripheral veins is unfeasible due to thrombus [1, 2]. Besides history-taking and clinical evaluation, patients should undergo duplex imaging followed by CT angiography performed to provide anatomic details for planning arterial reconciliation if necessary. Upon admission, the patient should be started on a broad spectrum of antibiotics since infection is polymicrobial with or without a fungus present. Patients with mycotic pseudoaneurysms due to intravenous drug abuse are uncommon, and the optimal management is uncertain; reported results are from a small retrospective case series. The contemporary treatment options include:

S. S. Hans, *Contemporary Management of Lower Extremity Aneurysmal Disease*,
https://doi.org/10.1007/978-3-032-00159-7_10

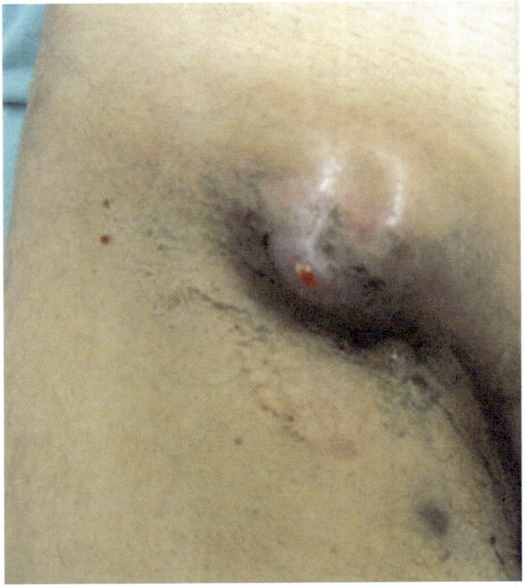

Fig. 10.1 Infected femoral artery pseudoaneurysm in a patient with IV drug abuse

1. Excision and debridement with ligation of the common femoral artery without revascularization
2. Excision and debridement with routine or selective revascularization

Reddy et al., in a landmark study, reported 54 cases of femoral artery pseudoaneurysms due to intravenous drug abuse and classified the patients into two groups [3].

Group A: Isolated involvement of common, superficial, or deep femoral artery
Group B: Involvement of common femoral artery bifurcation

Group A patients were treated by aneurysm ligation and excision, whereas Group B patients underwent excision and triple arterial ligation with or without vascular reconstruction. In Group A, no patients needed amputations. In Group B, 33% of patients who underwent ligation alone without revascularization required major amputation [3].

After complete evaluation, surgery is performed using suprainguinal (LLQ) oblique incision, exposing external iliac artery in the retroperitoneal plane, and a silastic vessel loop is passed. Another vertical incision is made directly over the pseudoaneurysm. If distal control is challenging, the aneurysm is opened, and intraluminal control is obtained by either a No. 4 or No. 5 Fogarty catheter or by Garrett arterial dilators [1]. Most authors report a 25%–35% rate of major amputation following aneurysm ligation and excision [2, 4, 5].

Options for Revascularization

After ligation of the femoral artery and extensive debridement of the soft tissues, revascularization may need to be performed. There are various options with difficult conduits for revascularization. These options include:

1. Use of superficial femoral-popliteal vein
2. Use of internal iliac artery
3. Extraanastomotic bypass, obturator bypass, or lateral bypass using PTFE or rifampin-impregnated Dacron graft

Harvesting of Superficial (SF) and Popliteal Vein

The incision is made over the lateral border of the sartorius muscle in the ipsilateral thigh to avoid infected tissue in the femoral triangle. Prior to harvesting of the SFV-popliteal vein, the infected site is covered with iodine-impregnated incision drape (3M™ Ioban™2 3M™ Health Care, St. Paul, MN) [5]. Following the exposure of the SF/PV, the side branches are ligated. The vein is harvested from the femoral area to just above the knee, and the larger side branches should be suture ligated. The ties are applied in close apposition to the vein wall because close apposition of the ligatures helps to reinforce the thin area with adventitia and periadvential tissue if present. The vein is then harvested, and its valves are lysed using Leather (Modified Mills) retrograde valvulotome (Becton, Dickinson, Franklin Lakes, NJ). The graft is placed in a cold heparinized saline solution with papaverine [4]. The SFA and the profunda femoris arteries are exposed and mobilized using the same incision extending to the anterior superior iliac spine with medial retraction of the sartorius muscle. If the SFA has any chronic occlusion, the harvested vein is anastomosed to the profunda femoris. The thigh incision is closed in layers. Resection and debridement of the mycotic aneurysm involving femoral artery and main branches are then performed with ligation of the proximal and distal portion of the artery.

Use of Internal Iliac Artery

In patients with mycotic aneurysms due to intravenous drug abuse, the great saphenous vein (GSV) is usually not available for autologous reconstruction as the superficial veins are often used for repetitive injections. Despite its short length, an interposition graft of the internal iliac artery has been used [1]. Its advantages include harvesting from a noninfected area with good size match and less prone to late aneurysmal dilatation. Harvesting of the internal iliac artery, however, requires laparotomy.

Use of Synthetic Grafts Routed Laterally or via Transobturator Route

If ligation of mycotic aneurysm results in severe ischemia of the LE with absent Doppler arterial flow in the foot, synthetic graft can be used via a transobturator route or laterally over the iliac crest.

Obturator Bypass Obturator bypass is an option for patients following debridement and ligation of the femoral artery. The proximal external iliac artery is exposed using a left flank retroperitoneal incision. The incision starts lateral to the rectus abdominus, midway between the umbilicus and symphysis pubis, and curves laterally upward to the external oblique muscle, and the fascia is incised in the direction of its fibers. After division of the internal oblique muscles and the transverse abdominus muscles, the peritoneal envelop is mobilized medially from the medial side of iliac crest, making certain that the plane of dissection is anterior to the iliopsoas fascia. The iliac artery bifurcation is exposed and mobilized, and silastic vessel loops are passed. The obturator membrane is exposed by palpating the pubis and is divided by Metzenbaum scissors with finger guidance. An 8 mm interring PTFE (WL Gore, Newark, DE) graft or deep vein is harvested as a conduit (SF and popliteal vein) and is anastomosed proximally to the distal common iliac artery or the proximal external iliac artery. A blunt-tipped tunneler (Gore or Garrett) is used from the obturator fascia into the medial thigh with distal anastomosis to mid- or distal SFA. The proximal anastomosis is performed prior to tunneling the graft into the thigh. If the situation is not an emergency, the SFV/popliteal vein should be harvested and used as an autologous conduit.

Passage of Graft Using the Lateral Route over the Iliac Crest

In some patients where there is considerable induration of the medial upper thigh due to inflammatory reaction, it is preferable for the graft (after completion of the proximal anastomosis) to be laterally over the iliac crest and then brought medially into a "C"-shaped configuration to be anastomosed to the proximal or the mid-SFA.

Exposure of the SFA in the Proximal Thigh

The sartorius is mobilized medially by incising the fascia along its lateral border following a skin incision parallel to the lateral border of the sartorius muscle. The dissection is done under the sartorius, and the muscle is retracted medially. The dissection plane is established between the vastus medialis and the adductor longus. The proximal SFA is dissected by careful sharp dissection. Silastic vessel loops are then passed. The deep femoral artery is exposed and mobilized by ligature and division of the lateral circumflex femoral vein crossing the artery.

Exposure of the SFA in the Middle Thigh

Skin incision is made in the middle of the thigh along the lateral border of the sartorius muscle. Dissection is performed in the Hunter's canal between the vastus medialis and the adductor longus muscle.

Many studies have reported that femoral mycotic aneurysms in patients with IV drug abuse should be managed by ligation and excision of the involved vessels with delayed revascularization when required. Most case series have shown that ligation of the femoral artery results in low incidence of amputation since there is significant amount of collateral flow due to repeated injury to the femoral artery. Some authors recommend checking the DP and/or PT artery Doppler signals, and if the signals are present, immediate revascularization is not mandatory.

Wound Management

Extensive debridement of infected site (artery and surrounding tissues) is performed with application of negative-pressure wound therapy (NWPT). Negative-pressure wound therapy gently pulls the fluid from the wound over time and helps reduce the edema and inflammation and aids in cleaning the wound. The wound usually heals by secondary intention. The use of negative-pressure wound therapy should be avoided in patients with exposed blood vessel. Negative-pressure wound therapy may sometimes result in increased bleeding from the wound bed. The common organisms cultured from mycotic femoral artery aneurysms are *Staphylococcus aureus*, *Enterococcus faecalis*, *Staphylococcus epidermidis*, *Salmonella*, *E. coli*, and anerobic species. The most common fungal agent causing mycotic aneurysms is *Aspergillus fumigatus*. Most infectious disease experts recommend a 6-week course of antibiotics after removal of all infected tissue.

Case Example

In September 2009, a 74-year-old man underwent endovascular abdominal aortic aneurysm and left CIA aneurysm repair, by use of a Talent graft (Medtronic, Dublin, Ireland) with an Amplatzer occluding plug at the origin of the left internal iliac artery (Fig. 10.2). Postoperative CTA showed a type III endoleak (Fig. 10.3). Attempted relining of the left iliac limb was unsuccessful, and the graft was converted to an aorto-uni-iliac graft configuration using three AneuRx cuffs, and a crossover femoral-femoral graft (using 8 mm PTFE INTERING®) was performed. The patient had a deep infection in the groin with involvement of the common femoral artery. Ten days later, the patient was taken back to the operating room, and a new 8 mm graft in a different tunnel was performed. The original femoral-femoral graft was removed, and an 8 mm graft was sutured end-to-end to the graft, which

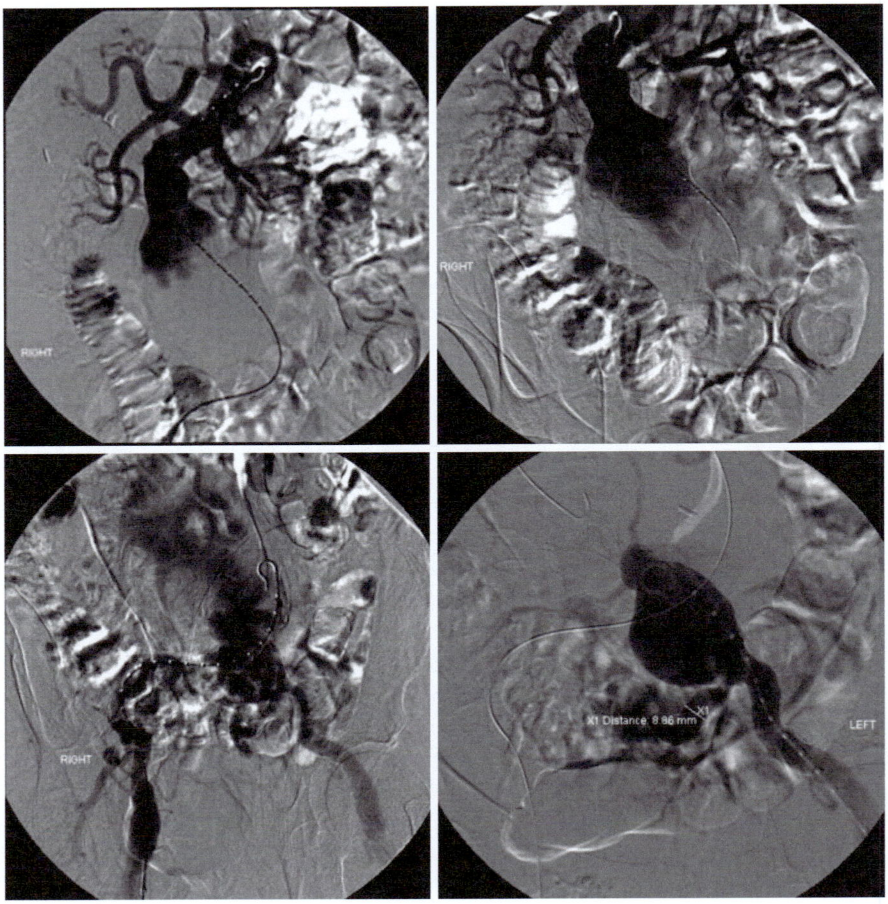

Fig. 10.2 Aortogram showing large AAA and left common iliac artery aneurysm and left hypogastric artery Amplatzer occlude plug placement

was placed a week earlier. This graft was anastomosed to the mid-superficial femoral artery in the subsartorial canal (Fig. 10.3). A sartorius myoplasty was performed, and the left groin healed following the application of the wound vacuum. A follow-up CTA showed no evidence of an endoleak with patent crossover femoral-femoral graft (Fig. 10.4). The patient died 14 months later following EVAR from congestive heart failure.

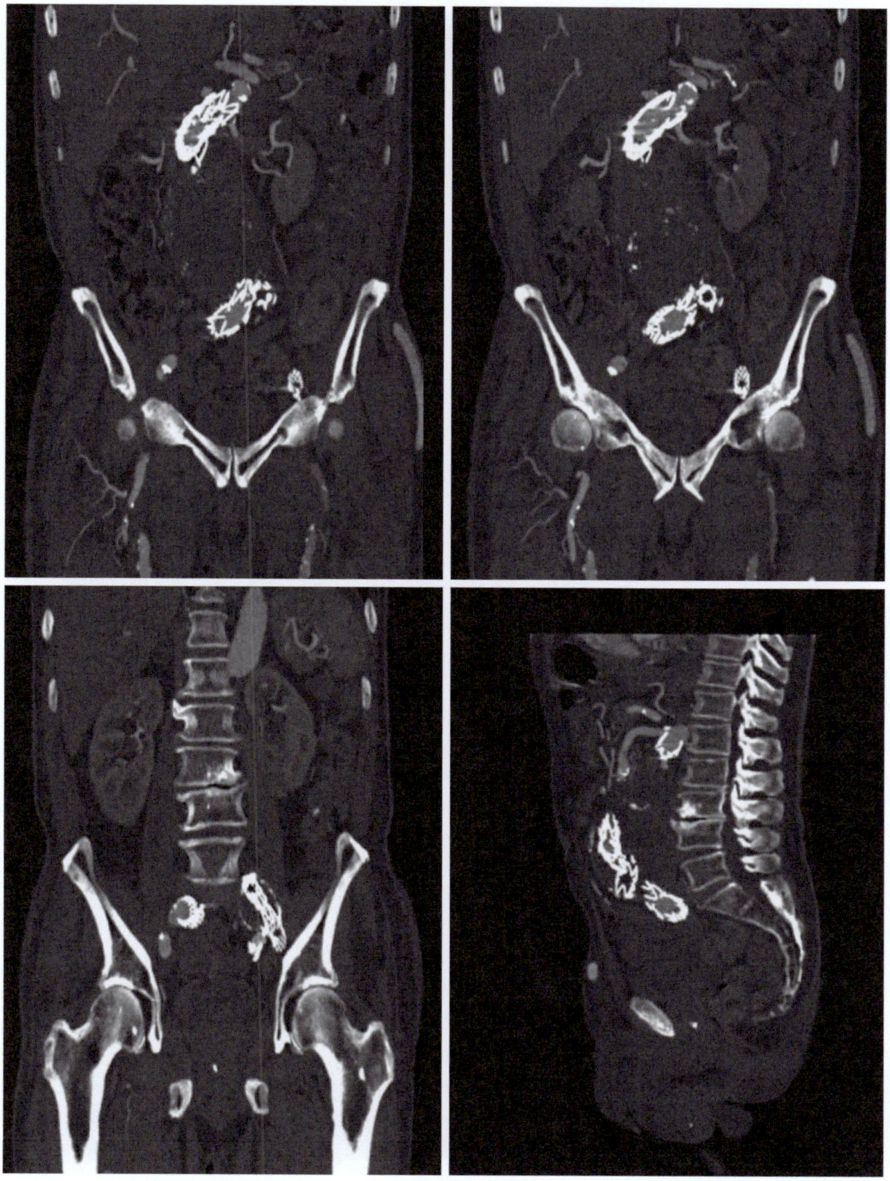

Fig. 10.3 CTA abdomen and pelvis showing type III endoleak

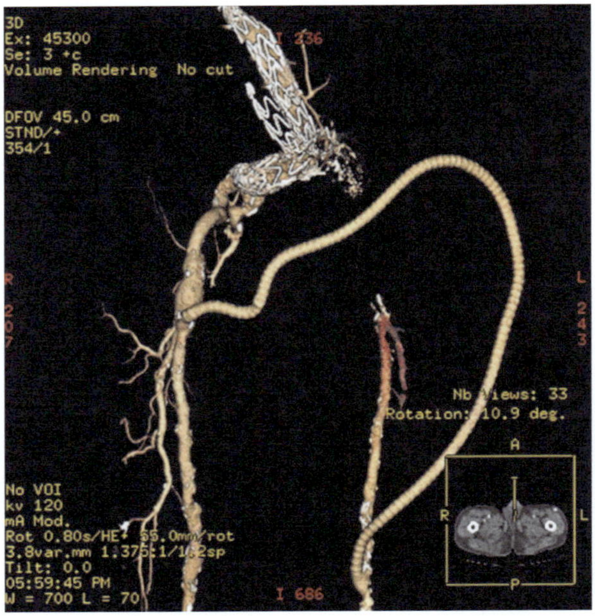

Fig. 10.4 CTA showing patent aorto-uni-iliac graft and a patent crossover femoral graft to mid-superficial femoral artery using anterolateral tunnel configuration

Invited Commentary

Daniel J. Reddy, MD, FACS

This chapter is a thorough and comprehensive review of an uncommon, but not rare, challenge to the vascular surgeon. A high-quality management outcome depends on the surgeon's mastery of requisite operative skills and also a firm grasp of the guiding principles of judgment, timing, and perseverance. These cases are often among the most challenging. The author has provided us with a lucid, detailed, and comprehensive review of this subject. This review will serve well the consultant surgeon both at the bedside and in the operating room.

Additional observations may help. Comorbid confounding variables often limit the treatment choices. These are extensive, sometimes life-threatening, rapid anaerobic progressive tissue destruction, overwhelming septic thrombophlebitis, and chronic lymphatic with advanced tissue edema. I have also encountered unexpected broken needles ("sharps") which pose a serious risk to the operating team. Intercurrent hepatitis C and/or HIV need to be considered. Synthetic prostheses are not recommended in such morbid tissue milieu.

References

1. Klonaris C, Katsargyris A, Papapetrou A, Vourliotakis G, Tsiodras S, Georgopoulos S, Giannopoulos A, Bastounis E. Infected femoral artery pseudoaneurysm in drug addicts: the beneficial use of the internal iliac artery for arterial reconstruction. J Vasc Surg. 2007;45(3):498–504. https://doi.org/10.1016/j.jvs.2006.11.014. Epub 20070124. PubMed PMID: 17254738.
2. Arora S, Weber MA, Fox CJ, Neville R, Lidor A, Sidawy AN. Common femoral artery ligation and local debridement: a safe treatment for infected femoral artery pseudoaneurysms. J Vasc Surg. 2001;33(5):990–3. https://doi.org/10.1067/mva.2001.114212. PubMed PMID: 11331839.
3. Reddy DJ, Smith RF, Elliott JP Jr, Haddad GK, Wanek EA. Infected femoral artery false aneurysms in drug addicts: evolution of selective vascular reconstruction. J Vasc Surg. 1986;3(5):718–24. PMID: 3517387.
4. Bell CL, Ali AT, Brawley JG, D'Addio VJ, Modrall JG, Valentine RJ, Clagett GP. Arterial reconstruction of infected femoral artery pseudoaneurysms using superficial femoral-popliteal vein. J Am Coll Surg. 2005;200(6):831–6. https://doi.org/10.1016/j.jamcollsurg.2005.02.012. PubMed PMID: 15922192.
5. Saini NS, Luther A, Mahajan A, Joseph A. Infected pseudoaneurysms in intravenous drug abusers: ligation or reconstruction? Int J Appl Basic Med Res. 2014;4(Suppl 1):S23–6. https://doi.org/10.4103/2229-516x.140715. PubMed PMID: 25298938; PMCID: PMC4181127.

Endovascular Repair of Popliteal Artery Aneurysms

11

Although rare, with a prevalence of 7.39/100,000, popliteal artery aneurysms (PAAs) are the most common peripheral artery aneurysms and account for 70% of all those diagnosed. Most popliteal artery aneurysms occur in the proximal segment and mid-portion of the popliteal artery, which are most frequently detected in men (95%) and are often bilateral (49–54%) [1, 2]. Unlike AAA, the incidence of rupture of a popliteal aneurysm is extremely uncommon (1.4%). Most patients present with an asymptomatic pulsatile mass or a prominent popliteal pulse. Some are detected by imaging studies performed for other vascular pathologies; more than two-thirds of patients will develop limb ischemia to a varying degree during a 5-year surveillance [1, 2]. Severe limb ischemia due to aneurysmal thrombosis or distal embolization may be the first presentation of popliteal artery aneurysm. Due to the high prevalence of symptomatic complications leading to a heightened risk of limb loss (40%), an aggressive approach to the repair of these aneurysms is recommended [1, 2].

Most interventionists recommend a 2 cm diameter threshold for elective repair and repair in those with extensive mural thrombus within the aneurysm sac. The traditional approach to PAA repair has consisted of aneurysm exclusion and revascularization using those autologous saphenous veins [1, 2]. Advances in technology have created endografts that support the advantages of a minimally invasive approach, with a shorter length of hospital stay and a quicker recovery [1, 2]. Due to incorporation of dual antiplatelet therapy following endovascular repair, improved patency rates of 80% at midterm follow- up have been reported. Much of the current literature on the endovascular repair of PAAs relies on the use of the GORE VIABAHN graft (WL Gore, Newark, DE), a nitinol stent with an ultrathin (100 mm) inner lining of heparin-bonded expanded PTFE. Advantages of this endograft include its flexibility (with tolerance to knee flexion), its inner lining as a PTFE instead of an irregular stent material, and the present manufacture design involving a contoured proximal edge designed to minimize endpoint inflammation which can lead to stenosis [1, 2].

S. S. Hans, *Contemporary Management of Lower Extremity Aneurysmal Disease*,
https://doi.org/10.1007/978-3-032-00159-7_11

Sizing and Planning

The patient's suitability for endovascular repair requires:

A. Normal proximal and distal landing zones of at least 2 cm
B. The discrepancy of the diameter between proximal and distal landing zone of ≤1 mm
C. Vessel tortuosity <45 degrees
D. Aneurysm diameter of less than 5 cm to prevent kinking of the endograft: a displacement of the endograft
E. At least two-vessel runoffs in the calf
F. And a required minimum length of 20 mm of the normal popliteal artery proximal to the origin of the anterior tibial artery with a diameter of 4.5 mm or greater (infrageniculate popliteal artery) [1, 2]

Zaghloul et al., from the largest single-center analysis following endovascular popliteal aneurysm repair, observed that a single-vessel tibial runoff and coverage below the knee were predictors of poor outcome [3]. Young, active patients or those with occupations like carpentry or gardening are more prone to thrombosis of the endograft and should preferably be treated with exclusion of the aneurysm and bypass using an open technique.

The length of the artery to be treated is controversial. Treating the entire length of an SFA and popliteal artery increases the likelihood of endograft thrombosis, resulting in acute limb ischemia as the collateral vessels are covered. The more stent grafts used increases the number of overlap zones as well as the incidence of thrombosis and stent fracture [1, 4]. In practice, endograft should cover all aneurysmal and ectatic segments with proximal and distal landing zones of 2 cm, preferably using a single covered stent.

The preoperative preparation includes medical optimization and use of dual antiplatelet drugs (aspirin and clopidogrel) that are continued for 6 weeks post-procedure. If the patient is on warfarin or apixaban, dual therapy with aspirin is a good alternate; however, adding dual antiplatelet therapy to the patient's anticoagulation increases the risk of bleeding.

Technique

The access to the aneurysm is obtained by way of either ipsilateral/antegrade or contralateral/retrograde femoral artery. A 7 Fr. sheath using a 0.018″ guidewire permits the delivery of an 8-mm-diameter endograft, which allows safe passage of the sheath up and over the aortic bifurcation. This cannot be performed safely with the higher-profile sheaths required for delivery of larger diameter devices. In those situations, an antegrade approach from either ipsilateral CFA or proximal SFA (or these arteries of sufficient diameter to admit a larger diameter sheath) percutaneously or via cut-down is required. For a 9–13 mm endograft, a 9–12 Fr. sheath is required and a 0.035″ guidewire with cut-down in the groin area for exposure of distal CFA or proximal SFA.

Following sheath access to the SFA, intravenous heparin is administered by the anesthesia team to maintain an activated clotting time (ACT) between 250 and 300 s. Arteriography is performed to confirm the preoperative imaging findings. In patients with suspected thrombus at the landing zones, intravascular ultrasound (IVUS) should be used to ensure that the landing site is satisfactory. Knee flexion lateral angiographic views should be considered to determine the "hinge point" of the femoropopliteal segment a few centimeters above the knee joint. In a patient requiring multiple endografts for coverage of popliteal aneurysms, this hinge point area is avoided in the overlap zone to reduce the incidence of stent fracture and stent thrombosis. The 0.035″ or 0.018″ stiff wire is advanced under fluoroscope guidance so that its tip is in the proximal segment of one of the infrapopliteal arteries. The selected endograft should be oversized by 10–15% proximally and distally. The endograft should not be oversized more than 15% of normal artery diameter, and the graft should not be oversized by more than 1–2 mm to minimize the risk of infolding, which may result in early thrombosis of the endograft. In patients with associated significant femoropopliteal occlusive disease, the delivery system may not advance "bare back" because the PTFE jacket may tear with maldeployment of the endograft. Advancing the access sheath with its dilator through these stenotic segments first facilitates placement of the delivery system to its target location. Following the advancement of the delivery system, the sheath is retracted so that the endograft is clear of its tip. Deployment of the endograft is achieved by pulling on a PTFE suture that opens the constraining PTFE jacket from around the device. Deployment should be performed under fluoroscopy so that radiopaque markers are in the desired locations, using gentle continuous traction in the PTFE suture to minimize device deflection. Deployment is from distal to proximal direction as the PTFE suture is removed with a slow but continuous traction. Vigorous tension on the PTFE suture may result in the bowing of the tip of the delivery system with resulting deployment within the aneurysmal segment—the so-called bowstring phenomenon.

If multiple endografts are used, the smaller device is placed first distally, and an overlap of 2–3 cm is maintained between them. Molding with an angioplasty balloon up to the diameter of the native artery is performed for the first device before deploying the second device. In the overlapping segments, the balloon is kept within the endograft to prevent arterial dissection of the adjacent native artery.

Completion arteriography is performed with the sheath injection to detect distal embolization, endoleaks, or any other abnormality such as kinking that impedes distal arterial flow. If a type I endoleak is detected proximally, further prolonged inflation with an angioplasty balloon should be performed, or an additional appropriately sized endograft can be used for proximal extension. Imaging should be considered with the knee in flexion and in extension to make certain that there is no kink in the endograft.

Follow-Up

Postoperative surveillance should be performed by duplex ultrasound (US) imaging at 6 weeks and every 6 months for the first 2 years. A two-view x-ray of the knee in extension and flexion to detect endograft migration, stent fracture, and kinking in the endograft should be performed [1, 2, 4]. The most common complications following endovascular repair are stent thrombosis, infection, and endoleak. With the use of dual antiplatelet therapy in the postoperative period, 5-year patency of 80% has been reported. Catheter-directed thrombolysis is effective in restoring patency of these endografts with reported secondary patency rates of 90–100% at 12 months and 80–90% at 24 months. In patients with type II endoleak with sac expansion, US-guided thrombin injection into the sac, or percutaneous coil embolization, should be considered. If ineffective, an open surgical approach can be performed by opening the sac of the feeding arteries with suture ligation [1, 2]. Type III endoleaks are treated by relining of the endograft [1, 2]. The reported incidence of graft occlusions was 38.5% in the stent fracture group versus 24.6% in the group without stent fracture [2, 4]. However, there was no difference between the two groups in terms of long-term patency rate. Multiple stent grafts and younger patient age were independent predictors of stent graft fracture. Stent graft thrombosis may be present with symptoms of acute ischemia or the patient may be asymptomatic or have minimal symptoms [1, 2].

Case Example

In April 2008, a 64-year-old male was seen in the outpatient clinic for evaluation of bilateral popliteal artery aneurysms, which measured 2.1 × 2.2 cm on the left and 2.5 × 2.7 cm on the right by duplex ultrasound with small amount of thrombus. The patient underwent left popliteal aneurysm exclusion using an 8 mm × 12 cm heparin-bonded GORE™VIABAHN™ Endoprosthesis graft (W.L. Gore, Newark, DE) using an 8 Fr. sheath (55-cm-long Cordis sheath) (Fig. 11.1).

In May 2008, the patient underwent exclusion of the right popliteal artery aneurysm with two overlapping GORE™VIABAHN™ Endoprosthesis stents each (8 mm × 15 cm long) since there was type I B endoleak following the deployment of the first covered stent. The patient underwent follow-up duplex imaging in June 2008, which showed patent-covered stents with satisfactory exclusion of popliteal aneurysm but with a 30% edge (lower end) stenosis at the stent and native popliteal artery junction on the right side.

In June 2015, the patient had a drop in the ankle brachial index (ABI) on the right side from 1.0 to 0.78. Arteriography showed 60% stenosis of the proximal end of the stent graft on the right involving superficial femoral artery with type I A endoleak, which was corrected by right superficial artery angioplasty and placement of a 9 mm × 4 cm self-expanding stent.

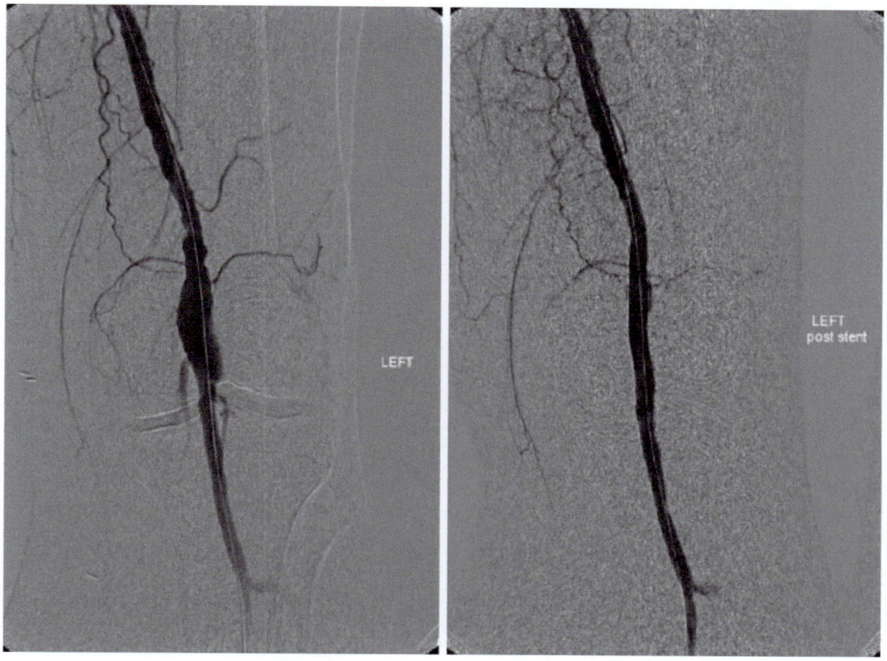

Fig. 11.1 Endovascular repair of the left popliteal aneurysm

In November 2018, the patient underwent right medial unicompartmental arthroplasty of the knee for degenerative arthritis that was unresponsive to conservative treatment. A review of the operative records shows that a tourniquet was applied to the mid-thigh. The patient came to the outpatient clinic in December 2018, with pain in the right lower extremity associated with paresthesias, with absent Doppler flow in the PT or DP artery. He was taken to the endovascular suite for arteriography and was found to have thrombosis of the entire distal and mid-superficial femoral artery, as well as the popliteal artery extending to the tibial peroneal trunk with thrombosis of the GORE™ VIABAHN™ Endoprosthesis stent graft (Fig. 11.2). Thrombolysis was started with an infusion catheter with occluding wire using bolus dose of 4 mg of TPA followed by 0.5 mg/h for 24 h. The patient was monitored in intensive care unit with partial lysis of the thrombus within 12 h. After 36 h, there was almost complete lysis because of 70% stenosis proximal and distal to the previously placed GORE™ VIABAHN™ Endoprosthesis stent; a covered stent extension of proximal 8 mm, diameter 5 cm long, and distal 8 mm × 2.5 cm GORE™ VIABAHN™ Endoprosthesis stent was performed (Fig. 11.3). Post-stent angioplasty was performed (Fig. 11.4). The procedure was performed through 7 F sheath (45-cm-long Pinnacle sheath). Later, the patient was found to have patent distal popliteal artery with a two-vessel runoff (posterior tibial and anterior tibial) and

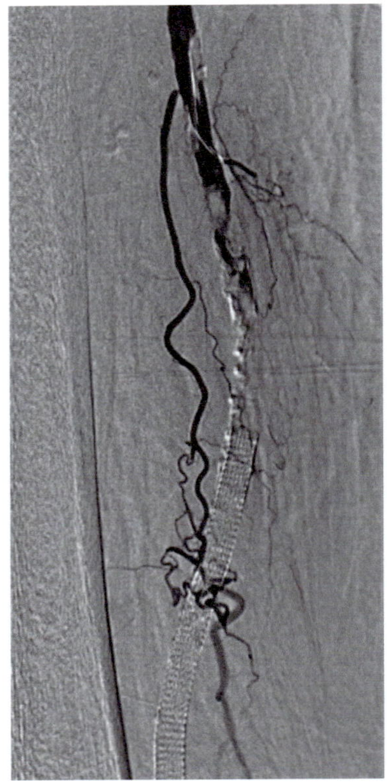

Fig. 11.2 Arteriogram showing the thrombosed right popliteal stent graft

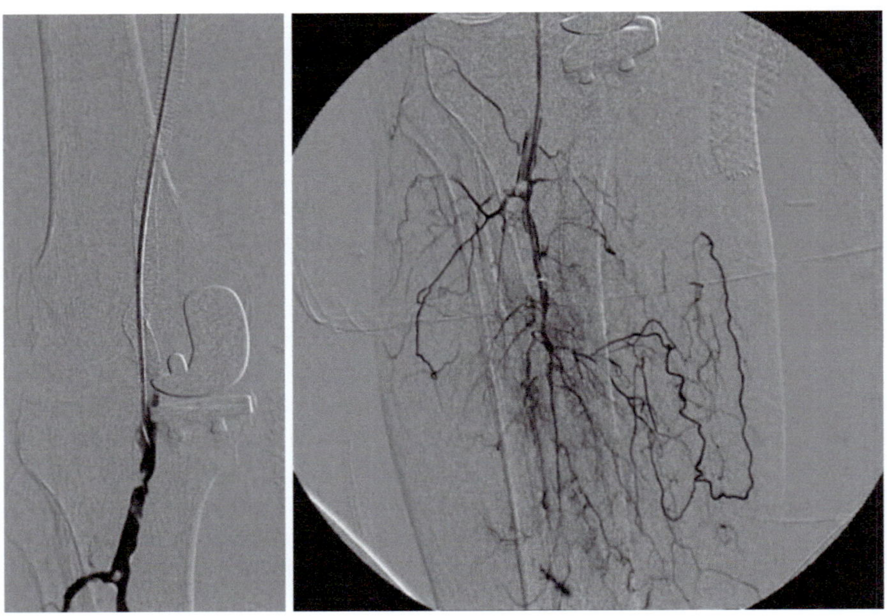

Fig. 11.3 Thrombolysis of the popliteal stent graft with infusion catheter in the distal popliteal artery and tibioperoneal trunk

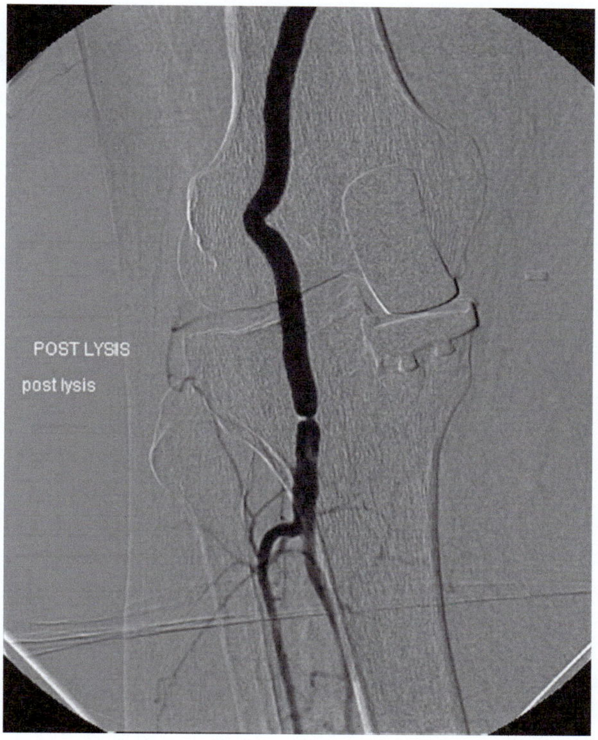

Fig. 11.4 Stenosis at the distal end of the stent graft

peroneal artery occlusion (Fig. 11.5). The patient developed posterior compartment hematoma in the right calf associated with severe pain most likely due to perforation of a muscular branch from the GLIDEWIRE. Fasciotomy of the posterior compartment (superficial and deep) was performed via a medial incision in the medial side of the calf. Evacuation of the hematoma and wound vac was applied. The patient had complete healing in 3 weeks, and he was followed by clinical exam and duplex/Doppler studies. He was last seen in October 2019 with normal ABIs on both sides, and duplex imaging showed satisfactory exclusion of the popliteal aneurysms.

Subsequently, the patient developed intractable congestive heart failure in 2021 and expired in February 2023 from persistent acute heart failure with associated renal failure.

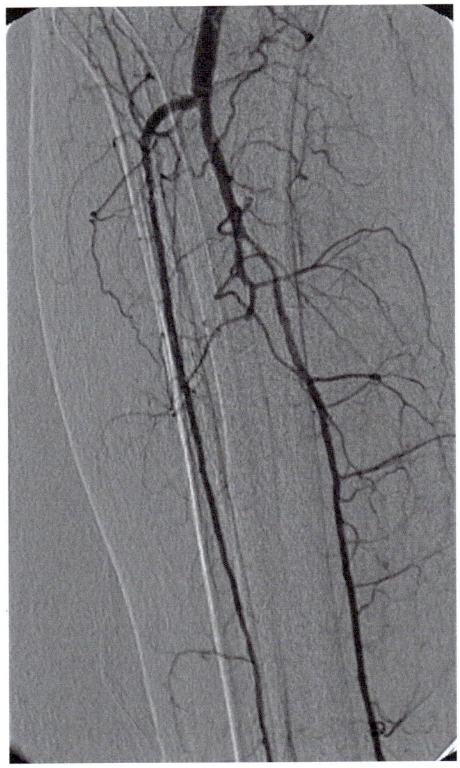

Fig. 11.5 Arteriography showing patent distal popliteal artery with two-vessel runoff (posterior tibial and anterior tibial) and peroneal artery occlusion

Invited Commentary

Raghu Motaganahalli, MD, RPVI, FRCS, FACS, DFSVS

The chapter on endovascular repair of popliteal aneurysms provides an excellent overview of the technique and evolving literature in the management of popliteal aneurysms. The treatment algorithm for popliteal aneurysm management is confounded by the indication and choice of intervention. The initial step in management should always be identifying if the patient even requires an intervention. Occasionally, patients may present with compressive symptoms such as deep venous thrombosis as the first symptoms besides others discussed in the chapter. Our guidelines based on the data, some of which is provided in this chapter, support treatment for aneurysms greater than 2 cm. As we have learned in our own practice, this is not always an easy answer. Our decision is guided by the patient's age, associated comorbidities, symptom status, and the morphology of the popliteal aneurysm that also play a significant role in this decision. Treatment decision can be influenced by the presence of the aortic aneurysm and how this may impact the future interventions. For patients deemed high surgical risk, it is recommended that repair be done at 3 cm or greater. As we continue to study this difficult topic, we will learn more about the relationship between size and symptom status but also about the degree of thrombus burden within these aneurysms and how this might affect future guidelines and clinical practice. Indeed, those patients with single-vessel outflow within the infrapopliteal vessels would not be a suitable candidate for endovascular repair for the risk of stent thrombosis and progression to limb threatening ischemia regardless of their surgical fitness. If they are asymptomatic and their surgical risk is prohibitive, conservative management and close surveillance might be the safer option in these patients.

Although we typically prefer open repair for good surgical candidates and younger patients, the advent of endovascular technology has afforded us the ability to care for patients who might otherwise have been managed medically. If adequate proximal and distal seal zone exist, as well as good inflow and minimum two-vessel outflow, endovascular repair can be an attractive option for repair. Careful procedural planning is critical to the success of endovascular repair of popliteal aneurysms. Inflow anatomy, aneurysm morphology, and outflow anatomy are all essential aspects to evaluate when planning a successful repair. As can be seen often, aneurysm disease is not always confined to the P2 segment of the popliteal artery. Degeneration can also be seen within the P1 segment or within the superficial femoral artery. Sizing for selection of the appropriate stent graft is vital. If available, imaging software to obtain a good centerline reconstruction should be employed. As mentioned, often the popliteal artery tapers to a healthier vessel within the P3 segment requiring a smaller diameter stent graft. While it is desirable to repair the aneurysm with a single stent, it is not always the case due to variation in the diameter of the proximal and distal stent attachment sites. The repair should begin with stent deployment in the distal popliteal artery and, then if necessary, extending into the larger diameter segments more proximally with distal overlap into the distal stent graft. Treatment planning should include choosing an appropriate size stent with a gradual escalation of the stent diameter as one progresses toward more proximal arterial system. In addition, a careful consideration should be given to having adequate overlapping of more than 2–3 cm especially in the large aneurysms, tortuous course of femoral and popliteal aneurysms to prevent a type 3 endoleak. Post-procedure, we recommend a regimen of dual antiplatelet therapy, typically for 3 months prior to consideration on transitioning to a single agent. As with any revascularization, surveillance with duplex imaging should be done routinely for stent patency as well as residual aneurysm sac expansion.

References

1. Hothem Z, Long GW. Endovascular repair of popliteal artery aneurysms. In: Hans SS, editor. Endovascular and open vascular reconstruction: a practical approach. Boca Raton: CRC Press; 2017. p. 69–73.
2. Aranson N, Ta M. Complications of stent graft for popliteal aneurysms. In: Hans SS, Conrad MF, editors. Vascular and endovascular complications: a practical approach. Boca Raton: CRC Press; 2021. p. 89–95.

3. Zaghloul MS, Andraska EA, Leake A, Chaer R, Avgerinos ED, Hager ES, Eslami MH. Poor runoff and distal coverage below the knee are associated with poor long-term outcomes following endovascular popliteal aneurysm repair. J Vasc Surg. 2021;74(1):153–60. PMID:33347999
4. Tielliu IF, Zeebregts CJ, Vourliotakis G, et al. Stent fractures in the Hemobahn/Viabahn stent graft after endovascular popliteal aneurysm repair. J Vasc Surg. 2010;51(6):1413–8. https://doi.org/10.1016/j.jvs.2009.12.071.

Open Repair of Popliteal Artery Aneurysm

12

The primary objective in the repair of popliteal artery aneurysms (PAAs) is the exclusion of the aneurysm from the circulation to prevent complications such as thrombosis or distal embolization. The standard approaches for repair of a PAA include both medial and posterior approaches [1, 2].

Medial Approach

The advantages of the medial approach include its familiarity to most vascular surgeons and its versatility in allowing for proximal and distal exposure in patients with involvement of the SFA and infrapopliteal artery being the distal arterial target for the bypass. Genicular arteries arising from the popliteal aneurysmal segment require suture ligation. They have the potential to retrogradely perfuse the excluded aneurysmal sac. For the medial approach, the patient is positioned supine, with the leg slightly externally rotated with a bump placed under the knee. The size of the bump depends on the size of the lower extremity. A larger bump is required in patients with a larger-sized lower extremity.

A medial incision is made above the knee to expose the popliteal artery longitudinally over the adductor tubercle represented by slight depression between the vastus medialis above and the sartorius below. If the GSV is needed, the incision can be made 2.0 cm posteriorly. After incision in the skin and subcutaneous tissues, the deep fascia is opened, followed by dissection in the medial intermuscular septum. The popliteal fossa is entered medially and anteriorly to the sartorius muscle. The proximal popliteal area can be palpated in the popliteal fat pad and is surrounded by venae comitantes and often intimately adherent to the popliteal artery. Exposure of the popliteal artery often requires division of the transverse branches of venae comitantes after ligature. During dissection, the saphenous nerve can be seen exiting the adductor hiatus and coursing superficially and inferiorly accompanying the GSV at or just below the knee. Every effort should be made to protect this nerve, but if there

S. S. Hans, *Contemporary Management of Lower Extremity Aneurysmal Disease*,
https://doi.org/10.1007/978-3-032-00159-7_12

is inadvertent injury to the nerve, division of the nerve resulting in numbness is often better tolerated than ongoing pain of a partially injured or entrapped nerve [1].

The medial exposure of the below knee segment of the popliteal artery is obtained by placing an incision posterior to the medial border of the upper tibia and anterior to the GSV and the incision placed slightly posteriorly if the GSV is to be used as a conduit. The fascia in the deep posterior compartment is opened, and a Weitlaner retractor is placed. The below knee segment of the popliteal artery is mobilized between the posterior tibial nerve and the popliteal vein. The origin of the soleus muscle from the soleus line is exposed, and its origin (tendons, white) fibers are divided with an electric cautery in an avascular plane. The anterior tibial vein crossing the popliteal artery at its bifurcation (into the anterior tibial artery (ATA) and tibioperoneal trunk) is exposed. A few other tributaries of the anterior tibial and the popliteal vein often require ligature and division using silver clips.

Further dissection of the aneurysm is performed to identify and ligate the genicular branches. The popliteal artery proximal and distal to the aneurysm is ligated. Arterial reconstruction is performed with either a reversed or non-reversed GSV with lysis of the valves (author's preference). The graft is tunneled anatomically or subcutaneously. In obese patients or in patients with difficult exposure due to a large aneurysm, the medial head of the gastrocnemius and tendons of the pes anserinus can be divided by electric cautery. The interposition graft is placed anatomically, following partial excision of the wall of the aneurysm with the suture ligature of the feeding arteries. If the graft is tunneled subcutaneously, it is advantageous to divide the below knee popliteal artery, and the distal anastomosis is performed end-to-end. This results in an anatomical course for the graft to follow since an end-to-side anastomosis may result in a kinking of the graft at the distal anastomosis with the potential of graft thrombosis. A completion arteriogram, or a duplex ultrasonography, should be considered prior to the closure.

Posterior Approach

The posterior approach is preferred for smaller aneurysms located at the knee joint line causing compressive symptoms. A lazy "S"-shaped incision with the patient in a prone position is started on the medial side of the lower thigh, extending laterally across the flexion crease of the knee and ending on the proximal position of the calf over the proximal small saphenous vein between the two heads of gastrocnemius muscle [1, 2]. The proximal part of the incision is used to expose the GSV, which can be harvested from the groin and upper thigh with the patient supine. After closing the incision, the patient is placed prone to continue the arterial reconstruction. Alternatively, if the SSV is large enough as visualized on preoperative venous mapping, the inferior segment of the incision can be extended, and the SSV can be harvested to be used as a conduit.

The neurovascular structure in the popliteal fossa including the popliteal artery is exposed [1, 2]. Dissection proceeds between the two heads of the gastrocnemius muscle staying medial to avoid injury to both the sural nerve and the small saphenous vein. As the two heads of gastrocnemius muscle are separated with the help of Weitlaner retractor, the nerve to the medial head of gastrocnemius will be encountered and may often need to be sacrificed in the distal exposure, but this does not result in any significant disability. Dissection proceeds medial to the popliteal vein and may require ligation of a few small branches to the popliteal vein. This exposure allows mobilization of the popliteal artery proximally from the adductor hiatus and distally to the bifurcation of the popliteal artery. The aneurysm is isolated as well as the normal- appearing popliteal artery proximally and distally to the aneurysm. Tourniquet inflation in the thigh proximal to the incision following exsanguination of the distal LE with an Esmarch wrap is a satisfactory alternative technique. The aneurysm is opened longitudinally and is partially excised, and the selected bypass conduit is sutured in place with end-to-end anastomosis proximally and distally with 6″0″ CV polypropylene suture.

Results

The risk of amputation within 30 days is 1.4% in asymptomatic patients [3, 4]. An excellent 1-year patency rate of 96% with the use of saphenous vein versus 67% for those with prosthetic conduit has been reported [3, 4]. The posterior and medial approaches have been found to be of equal value.

Case Example 1

A 64-year-old man with a BMI of 37.75 was found to have bilateral large popliteal aneurysms. The right was 5.5 cm, and the left was 3.5 cm in diameter; the right popliteal artery aneurysm also had a large amount of thrombus. He had ischemic rest pain and numbness in the right foot. Doppler study showed ABI (0.5) and TBI (0.48) on the right. Arteriography showed thrombosed right popliteal aneurysm, with two-vessel runoff and retrograde flow to the popliteal artery through the collaterals (Figs. 12.1 and 12.2). The left popliteal aneurysm had partial thrombus but with satisfactory runoff. It was decided to perform open repair of the right popliteal aneurysm by partial excision and vein bypass using the medial approach.

An incision was made in the lower thigh to the upper calf on the medial side. Subcutaneous tissues were incised, and the great saphenous vein was preserved. The tendons of the pes anserinus and the medial head of the gastrocnemius were divided. A dissection plane in the septum between the vastus medialis and sartorius was opened, preserving the saphenous nerve. The popliteal aneurysm was exposed, and the proximal popliteal artery proximal to the aneurysm was mobilized between the two femoral veins accompanying the artery. The silastic vessel loop was passed, and the distal popliteal artery just proximal to the crossing of the anterior tibial vein was exposed. The patient was given 12,500 units (100 units/kg) of heparin. After application of the distal vascular clamp, the proximal vascular clamp was applied to the proximal popliteal artery after the silastic vessel loops had been passed. An

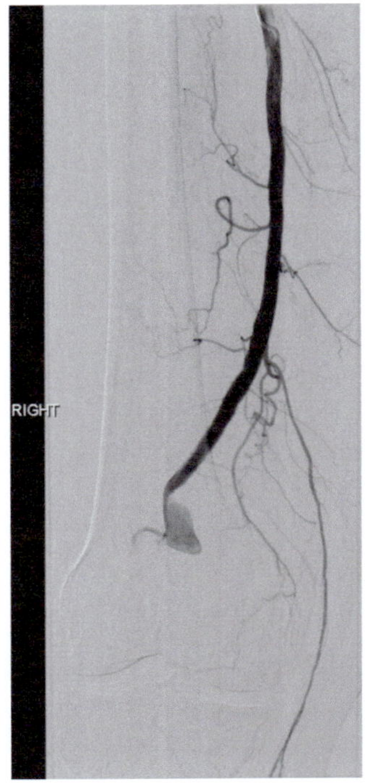

Fig. 12.1 Arteriogram showing the thrombosed right popliteal aneurysm

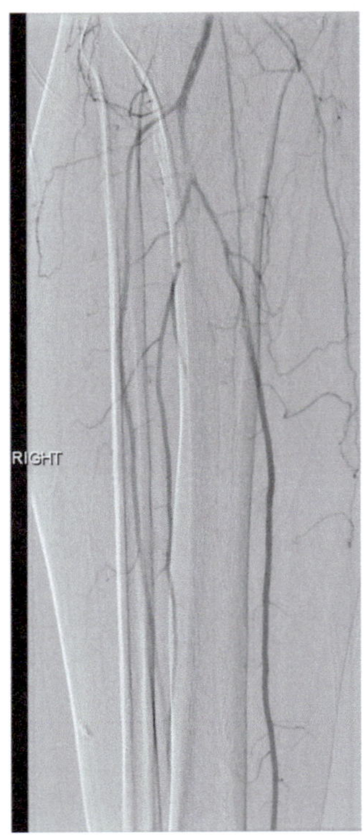

Fig. 12.2 Arteriogram showing retrograde filling of the tibioperoneal trunk via collaterals

incision over the aneurysm was made in its anterior wall (Fig. 12.3). A large amount of the thrombus was removed (Fig. 12.4). There was retrograde bleeding with pulsatile flow from the genicular arteries, which was controlled with figure-of-eight 4-0 cardiovascular polyprolene sutures. The greater saphenous vein was harvested from the upper thigh near the saphenofemoral junction to the mid-thigh using an oblique incision. All the side branches were ligated proximally, and silver clips were applied distally and then divided. The proximal end of the GSV was slit longitudinally, and a proximal anastomosis end-to-side to the proximal popliteal artery was performed using 6-0 cardiovascular Prolene running suture. The retrograde valvulotome was passed; valve leaflets were divided, and a pulsatile flow at the lower end of vein graft was observed. The anterior surface of the venous conduit is marked with indelible skin marking pen to avoid torsion or kinking of the graft. An end-to-end anastomosis with 6-0 cardiovascular Prolene running suture of the distal end of the vein to the distal popliteal artery was performed (Fig. 12.5). The wound was closed in layers. Ten weeks later, the patient underwent a partial excision and interposition GSV graft for the contralateral left popliteal aneurysm.

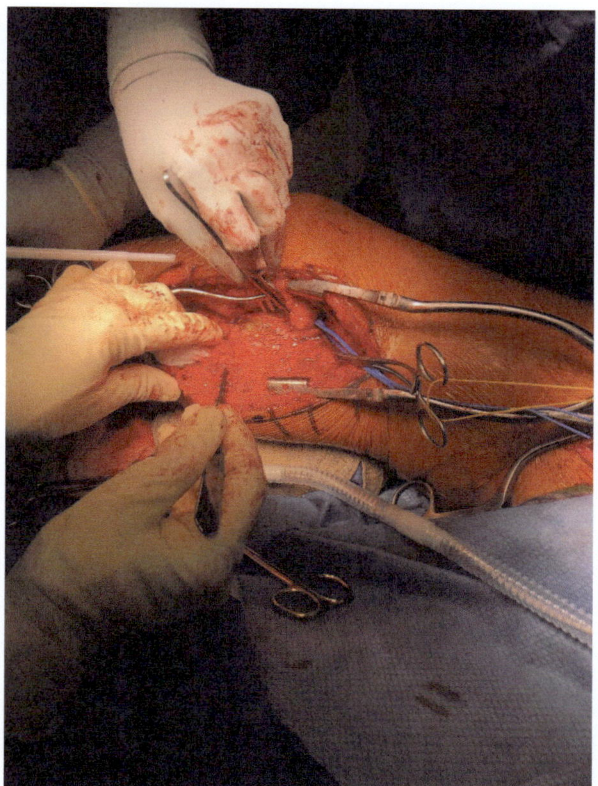

Fig. 12.3 Intraoperative photograph of the right popliteal aneurysm following incision in its anterior wall

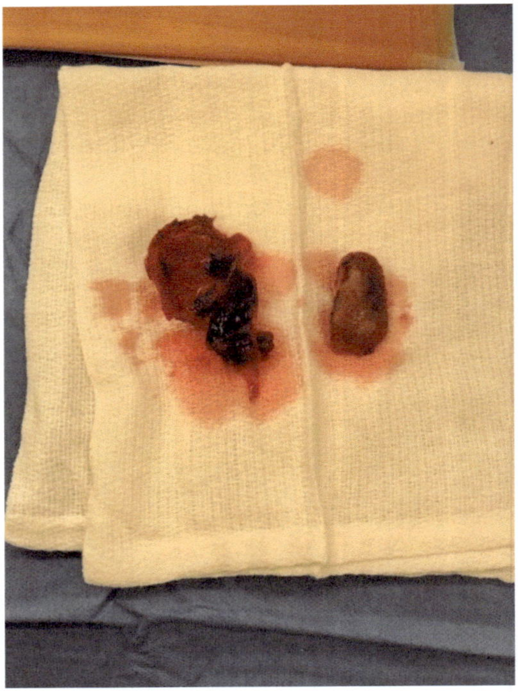

Fig. 12.4 Thrombus removed from the right popliteal aneurysm

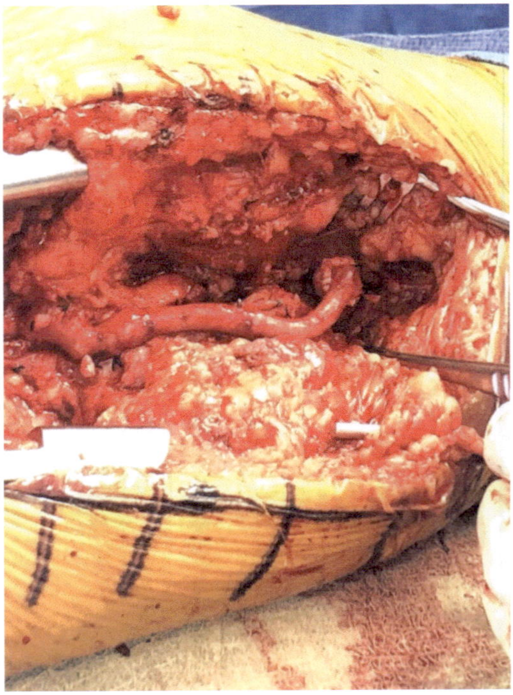

Fig. 12.5 Interposition GSV graft after partial excision of the large right popliteal aneurysm

Case Example 2

A 66-year-old man presented to the ER with a 2- to 3-day history of progressive pain in the right calf, with increasing severity and difficulty in ambulation. He had type 2 diabetes mellitus and hypertension. Computed tomography angiography (CTA) showed 4.5 × 3.7 × 3.8 cm popliteal aneurysm with a large amount of thrombus with diminished flow detected in infrapopliteal arteries consistent with monophasic Doppler artery signals in PT and DP arteries at the ankle (Fig. 12.6a, b). The great saphenous vein (GSV) was harvested from the right upper thigh in supine position using a posterior approach; aneurysm was opened; genicular branches were suture ligated; and an interposition GSV (Figs. 12.7 and 12.8) graft was performed, with successful restoration of blood flow to the lower extremity.

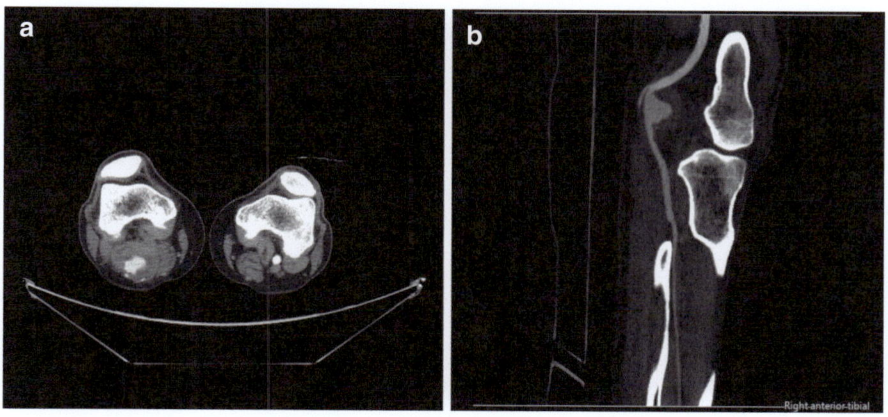

Fig. 12.6 (**a** and **b**) CTA with runoff showing the large right popliteal aneurysm with moderate to large amount of thrombus

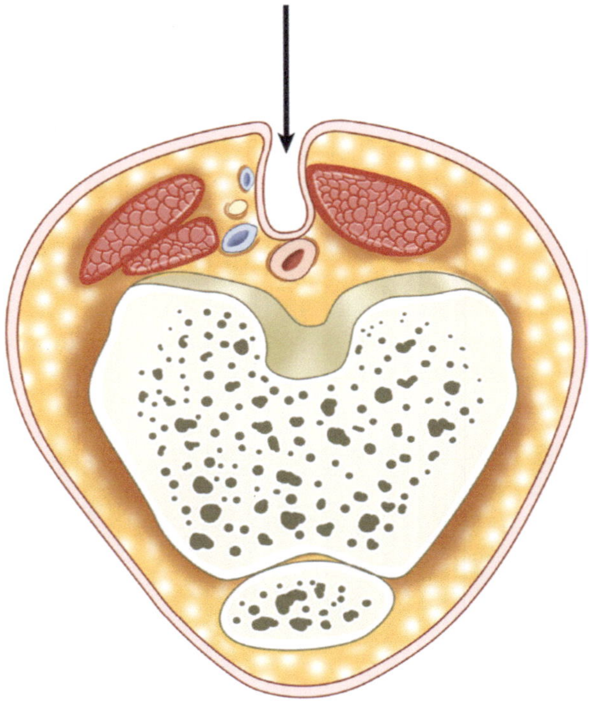

Fig. 12.7 Image demonstrating plane of dissection for posterior approach to popliteal artery, staying medial to the major nerves and veins

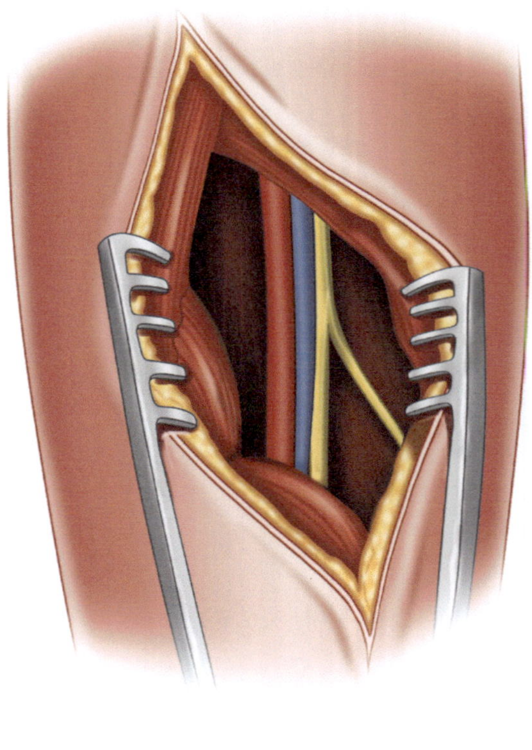

Fig. 12.8 Image demonstrating posterior exposure of the popliteal artery

Invited Commentary

Mitchell Weaver, MD, FACS

This chapter describes the operative treatment of popliteal artery aneurysms, which are the most common true peripheral artery aneurysms encountered by the vascular surgeon. Popliteal aneurysms are often associated with contralateral and extra-popliteal aneurysm. Popliteal artery aneurysms may be detected as an asymptomatic pulsatile mass on physical exam or noted as an incidental finding on an imaging study. However, it may also present with symptoms either acute or chronic. Acute symptoms include acute limb-threatening ischemia from popliteal artery thrombosis or thromboembolism or rarely secondary to rupture. Chronic symptoms include claudication or tissue loss, which usually have an insidious onset due to chronic silent embolization. Local compression of the nerve or vein may lead to pain and paresthesia or limb swelling.

The two approaches to repair the popliteal arteries described in this chapter include the posterior approach and the medial approach. The vascular surgeon must be familiar with both operations. The posterior approach has the advantage of a direct approach to the aneurysm and allows for complete excision of the aneurysm, which is beneficial when significant local compression symptoms are present. This approach requires the diseased aneurysmal artery be limited, usually from Hunter's canal proximally to the origin of the anterior tibial artery origin distally. A recent meta-analysis suggests superiority of the posterior approach over medial approach for patency, aneurysm exclusion, and need for reoperation [5]. The medial approach, on the other hand, is the most common approach reported. Advantages to this approach include its familiarity to most surgeons, the versatility it allows for proximal and distal exposure such as in cases of superficial femoral artery involvement or tibial artery target, as well as ready access to the great saphenous vein. With this approach, the artery is ligated proximal and distal to the aneurysm with interval bypass. Attempt is made as well to ligate side branches of popliteal artery, as there is risk of aneurysm sac growth if it remains pressurized from patent-preserved side branches, as unlike with the posterior approach, the aneurysm is not excised.

References

1. Weaver M. Popliteal aneurysm repair – primary and recurrent. In: Hans SS, Weaver MR, Nypaver TJ, editors. Primary and repeat arterial reconstructions. Cham: Springer; 2023. p. 153–62.
2. Hermann J, Johnson J, Oppat W. Open popliteal artery aneurysm repair. In: Hans S, Shepard A, Weaver M, et al., editors. Endovascular and open vascular reconstruction: a practical approach. Boca Raton: Taylor & Francis Group, LLC; 2017. p. 269–73.
3. Pulli R, Dorigo W, Troisi N, et al. Surgical management of popliteal artery aneurysms: which factors affect outcomes? J Vasc Surg. 2006;43(3):481–7. https://doi.org/10.1016/j.jvs.2005.11.048.

4. Huang Y, Gloviczki P, Noel AA, et al. Early complications and long-term outcome after open surgical treatment of popliteal artery aneurysms: is exclusion with saphenous vein bypass still the gold standard? J Vasc Surg. 2007;45(4):706–13.; discussion 13–5. https://doi.org/10.1016/j.jvs.2006.12.011.
5. Phair A, Hajibandeh S, Hajibandeh S, Kelleher D, Ibrahim R, Antoniou G. Meta-analysis of posterior versus medial approach for popliteal artery aneurysm repair. J Vasc Surg. 2016;64(4):1141–1150.e1.

13 Management of Mycotic Popliteal Artery Aneurysm and Popliteal Pseudoaneurysm

Mycotic aneurysms have been described in many arterial trees and may be present because of primary or secondary infection. Primary mycotic aneurysms of the popliteal artery are uncommon, and though initially thought to be due to a fungus infection, bacterial infection is now recognized as the most common cause. The common pathogens include *Staph epidermidis*, *Salmonella* species, *Campylobacter*, *S. aureus*, *Listeria monocytogenes*, *Strept pneumoniae*, *S. bovis*, *S. viridans*, *E. coli*, *Candida albicans*, and *Mycobacterium tuberculosis*. Most mycotic aneurysms infected with *S. epidermidis* have an indolent course, and isolation of *S. epidermidis* is often difficult [1–4].

Patient may present with a fever, knee pain, or with or without palpable tender mass in the popliteal fossa; untreated popliteal mycotic aneurysms may rupture. Lab data may show elevated white blood cell (WBC) count, sedimentation rate, and C-reactive protein. Blood culture is often positive; CT angiography, color-duplex sonography, and MR angiography are useful in the diagnosis and planning treatment. Recently, ^{18}F-FDG PET/CT detection of mycotic popliteal aneurysm has been reported with an intense focal update of the radioisotope.

Management

Following identification and treatment of the primary source of infection, the popliteal aneurysm is treated by complete excision and revascularization with an autologous graft. Endovascular repair with stent graft repair should be avoided but can be considered in an extremely high-risk patient presenting rupture as a bridge. For definitive repair of an autologous vein, using the great saphenous vein (GSV) or the deep veins (SFV/popliteal vein) is the conduit of choice. Failure of revascularization may result in major amputation of the lower extremity.

S. S. Hans, *Contemporary Management of Lower Extremity Aneurysmal Disease*,
https://doi.org/10.1007/978-3-032-00159-7_13

Popliteal Artery Pseudoaneurysms

Popliteal artery pseudoaneurysm are usually traumatic in origin; penetrating trauma is the most common cause, and many case reports have documented popliteal artery pseudoaneurysms due to blunt trauma. Pseudoaneurysms of the popliteal artery are more commonly encountered in military trauma: the reported incidence is less than 3.5% of all civilian popliteal aneurysms compared to 17.6% in World War II traumatic aneurysms, 27% in the Korean war, and 9.5% in the Vietnam war. Popliteal artery pseudoaneurysms after extreme hyperextension of the knee has been reported.

Following orthopedic operations (knee arthroplasty, osteotomy of knee), popliteal artery pseudoaneurysms are often encountered in patients presenting pain and discomfort in the popliteal fossa and calf together with associated swelling of the lower extremity [5, 6].

Color-flow duplex imaging is diagnostic, and CTA helps in defining the neck of the pseudoaneurysm and outflow vessels. This is best managed by the placement of a covered stent using contralateral femoral access (Figs. 13.1 and 13.2). Residual symptoms of pain, discomfort, and swelling may persist after endovascular intervention, but operative repair is usually not necessary.

The author recently encountered a large pseudoaneurysm 10 years following femoral popliteal bypass with non-reversed GSV at the popliteal anastomosis (Figs. 13.3 and 13.4). The patient was treated with a composite graft using an interposition PTFE graft (6 mm) anastomosed proximally to a vein bypass and distally to a below-the- knee popliteal artery (Figs. 13.5 and 13.6).

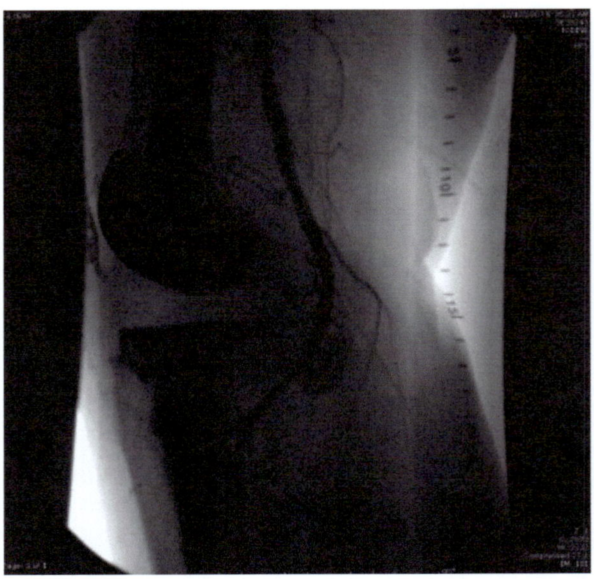

Fig. 13.1 Arteriogram via contralateral femoral approach showing the pseudoaneurysm of the right popliteal artery

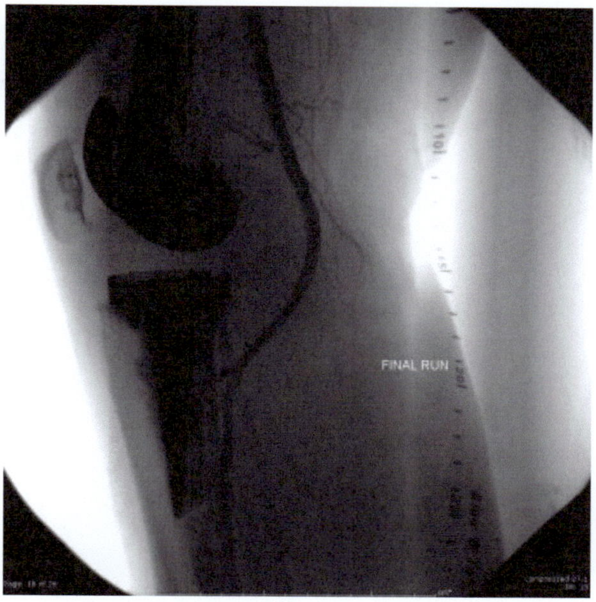

Fig. 13.2 Arteriogram showing the successful exclusion of the popliteal artery pseudoaneurysm

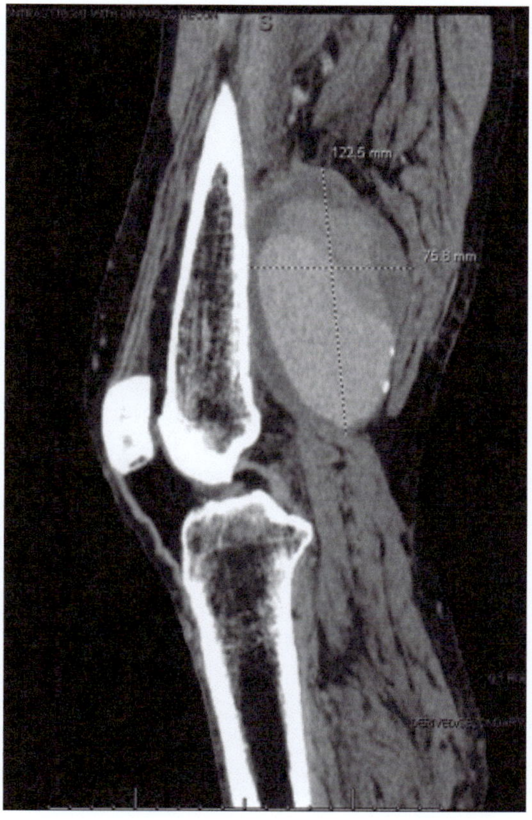

Fig. 13.3 CTA showing large right popliteal anastomosis following femoral popliteal bypass (vein)

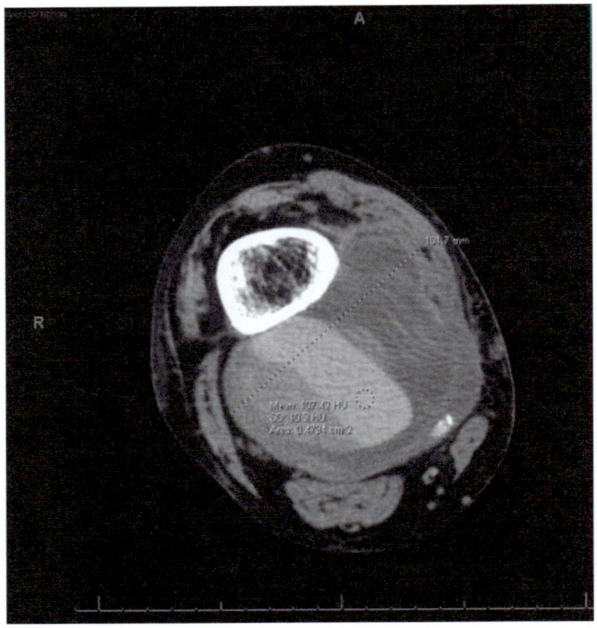

Fig. 13.4 CTA showing large right popliteal anastomosis following femoral popliteal bypass (vein)

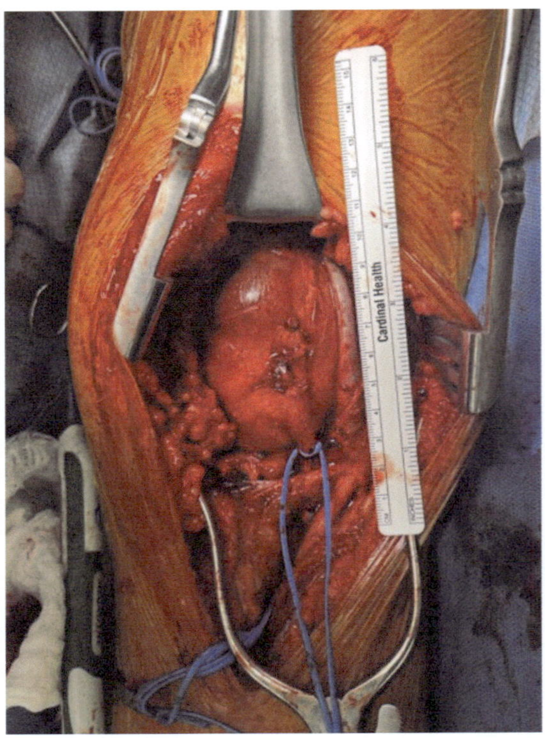

Fig. 13.5 Exposed popliteal anastomotic aneurysm using the posterior approach

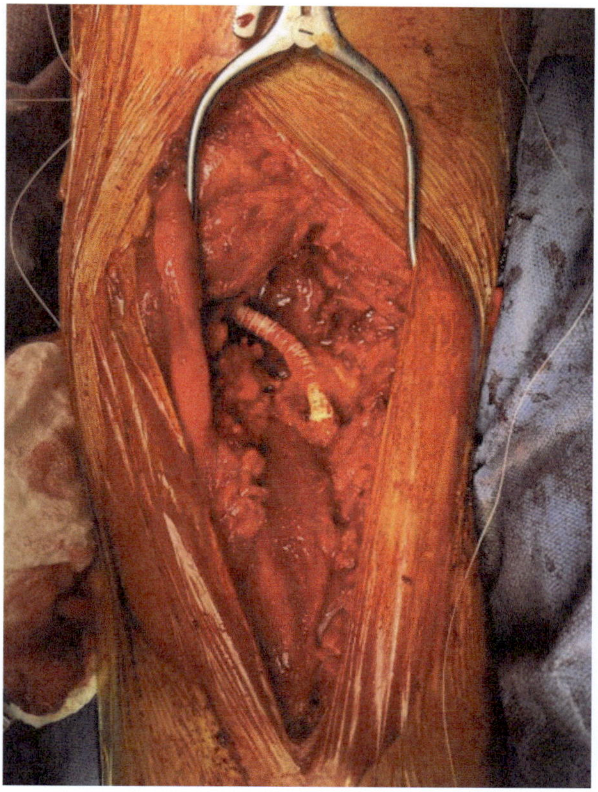

Fig. 13.6 PTFE graft anastomosed from vein graft (remote) to the distal popliteal artery

Case Example

A 54-year-old man came to the vascular clinic with complaints of pain in the left lower extremity from the knee to the foot. He was being treated for endocarditis of the prosthetic aortic valve with intravenous antibiotic. The patient had a Bentall procedure last June 2022; he presented to the vascular clinic with an ischemic left lower extremity and had palpable left femoral pulse, but popliteal posterior tibial and dorsalis pedis pulses were not palpable. The ankle-brachial index on the right was 0.96 and on the left was 0.59, with a toe-brachial index of 0.42 on the left.

On November 1, 2023, the patient underwent suction thrombectomy of the left popliteal artery and tibioperoneal trunk using 6F, 135-cm-long Rotarex atherectomy and thrombectomy device (BD-Becton Dickinson and Co., Franklin Lakes, NJ), followed by drug-coated balloon angioplasty of the left popliteal artery (Figs. 13.7 and 13.8) resulting in the restoration of the arterial flow with multiphasic signals in posterior-tibial and dorsalis pedis artery. A few days following arterial intervention, the patient developed increased swelling of the left lower extremity around the knee and upper calf. Duplex imaging revealed large aneurysms of the popliteal artery (Figs. 13.9 and 13.10). CTA demonstrated large left popliteal aneurysm with fat

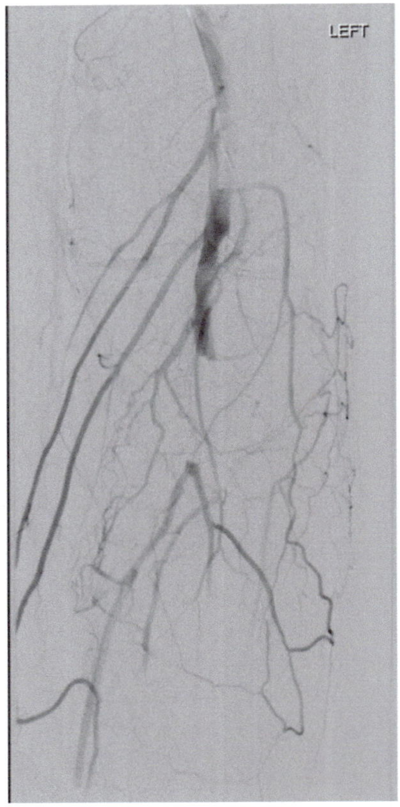

Fig. 13.7 Arteriogram showing the left popliteal artery occlusion

Fig. 13.8 Arteriogram showing the left popliteal artery following Rotarex and by drug-coated angioplasty

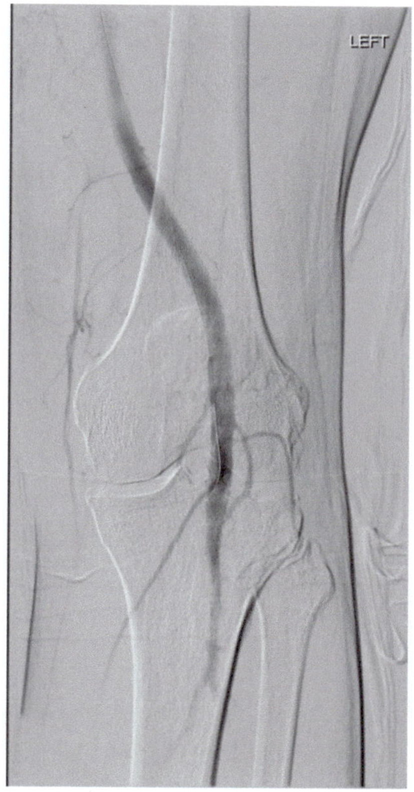

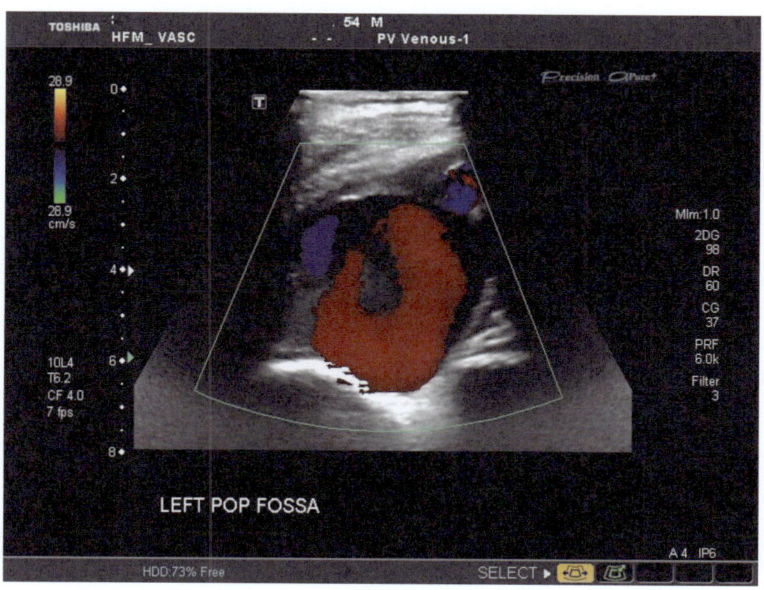

Fig. 13.9 Duplex imaging showing the large left popliteal artery aneurysm

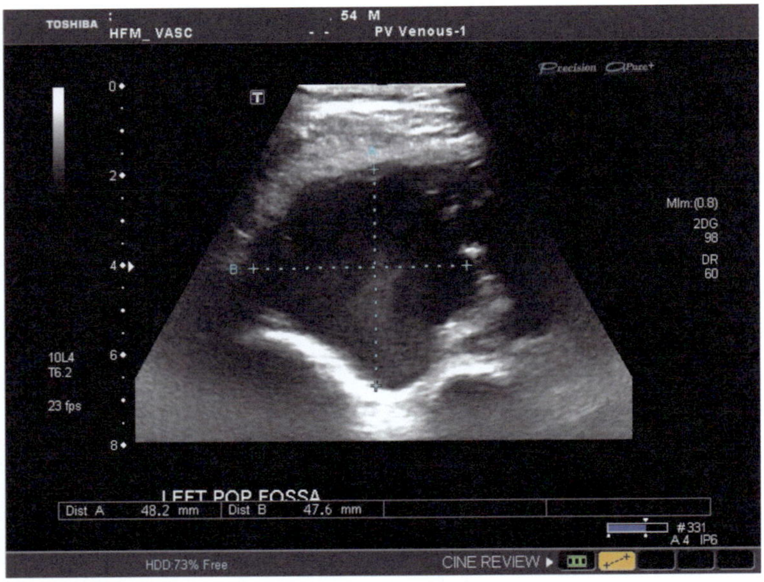

Fig. 13.10 Duplex imaging showing the large left popliteal artery aneurysm

stranding, indicating risk of impending rupture. On November 14, 2023, the patient was taken to the operating room (OR) on emergency basis, and the right great saphenous vein was harvested in a "frog-leg position." The patient was then placed prone, and using a lazy "s"-shaped incision, the proximal popliteal artery was exposed. A non-reversed interposition vein graft with lysis of the valve was anastomosed to the proximal popliteal artery and distally to the tibioperoneal trunk following resection of the mycotic aneurysms. The patient was continued on intravenous antibiotics, but he developed recurrent prosthetic valve endocarditis in December 2023 with *E. faecium* bacteremia. Transesophageal echocardiography (TEE) revealed a 2 cm mobile echodensity attached to the ventricular surface of the bioprosthetic valve. The source of the *E. faecium* bacteremia was thought to be colonic malignancy. A repeat TEE in February 2024 was suspicious for an abscess between the aortic valve and the aortic wall. In March 2024, the patient underwent a redo of the Bio-Bentall procedure (aortic root replacement) and (tissue valve graft: #29 Magna valve in #32 Gelweave Valsalva graft) via redo sternotomy. He was continued antibiotics, and at last follow-up, mild swelling and discomfort in the left calf were noted.

References

1. Lajos P, Bangiyev R, Safir S, et al. Mycotic popliteal artery aneurysm with rapid enlargement post-bypass. Cureus. 2021;13(6):e15746. https://doi.org/10.7759/cureus.15746.
2. Jolly K, Barratt R, Nair A. A rare case of Streptococcus sanguinis mycotic popliteal aneurysm. JMM Case Rep. 2014;1(4):e001479. https://doi.org/10.1099/jmmcr.0.001479.
3. Megalopoulos A, Siminas S, Trelopoulos G. Traumatic pseudoaneurysm of the popliteal artery after blunt trauma: case report and a review of the literature. Vasc Endovasc Surg. 2006;40(6):499–504. https://doi.org/10.1177/1538574406290037.
4. Woolgar JD, Reddy DS, Robbs JV. Delayed presentation of traumatic popliteal artery pseudoaneurysms: a review of seven cases. Eur J Vasc Endovasc Surg. 2002;23(3):255–9. https://doi.org/10.1053/ejvs.2001.1582.
5. Hans SS, Shepard AD, Reddy P, et al. Iatrogenic arterial injuries of spine and orthopedic operations. J Vasc Surg. 2011;53(2):407–13. https://doi.org/10.1016/j.jvs.2010.08.084.
6. Ge PS, Ishaque BM, Bonilla J. Popliteal artery pseudoaneurysm after isolated hyperextension of the knee. Ann Vasc Surg. 2010;24(7):950.e7–e11. https://doi.org/10.1016/j.avsg.2010.01.014.

Acute Thrombosis of the Popliteal Aneurysm

14

The acute symptoms of thrombosis are manifested in 28% of patients diagnosed with popliteal artery aneurysm (PAA). The manifestation of acute thrombosis is variable. Acute thrombosis may occur in a popliteal aneurysm which is localized in the knee area, or an acute thrombosis may occur in a diffusely aneurysmal superficial femoral and popliteal arteries; the aneurysmal diameter is usually not very large. In several patients, thrombosis of PAA may only result in symptoms of intermittent identification which tends to improve with conservative management. A significant number of patients with thrombosis of PAA present limb-threatening ischemia with either no sensory deficits or minimal sensory loss; in the absence of paralysis, it is defined as Rutherford Grade II A, while in the presence of sensory deficit, it extends to the toes and defined as Grade II B [1]. Rutherford Grade III limb ischemia presents with associated muscle paralysis of the lower leg, complete sensory loss, and absent Doppler signals in the foot. Most patients with thrombosed PAA and Rutherford Grade I ischemia do not need any intervention. Patients with Grade III ischemia most likely will need major amputation (below knee BK or above knee AK).

Patients with Rutherford Grade II A or B ischemia often present to the ER with a painful lower extremity associated with paresthesia and motor deficit, and if the ischemia is severe (Rutherford Grade II B), this is often associated with thromboembolic occlusion of the runoff vessels.

After obtaining patient history in the ER, a Doppler arterial study is performed, followed by a CTA of the abdominal aorta and a CTA series of the lower extremity. In patients presenting with an arterial occlusion due to thrombosed popliteal artery aneurysm, the prior history of intermittent claudication is absent, and the patient often has palpable pulses in the contralateral lower extremity. An astute clinician may be able to palpate a pulsatile mass in the contralateral popliteal fossa as 40–50% of popliteal artery aneurysms (PAAs) are bilateral.

The patient should be started on intravenous heparin drip, and an urgent arteriography should be obtained depending on the grade of the ischemia. A contralateral

S. S. Hans, *Contemporary Management of Lower Extremity Aneurysmal Disease*,
https://doi.org/10.1007/978-3-032-00159-7_14

femoral artery access is preferred. If the aneurysm is occluded and runoff vessels are patent, open repair (exclusion) and bypass are performed during the same admission. In the absence of visualization of any outflow vessel and in the patient with a Grade II A ischemia, catheter thrombolysis is started to restore flow into a potential target vessel in the calf. If the limb is immediately threatened (Rutherford Grade II B), the patient should be emergently taken to the hybrid operating room, and using a medial approach, the distal popliteal artery is exposed. The origin of the soleus muscle is taken down from the soleal line, and the anterior tibial vein crossing the popliteal artery bifurcation is exposed and is ligated on each side and divided. A longitudinal arteriotomy incision is made in the distal popliteal artery extending to the proximal tibioperoneal trunk, and a small Fogarty catheter (No. 2 or 3) is passed into each tibial artery to remove any thrombi. Occasionally, no clots can be retrieved whether due to very distal embolization or the laminated thrombus adherent to tibial and peroneal arteries. The author has encountered, in some patients, the only runoff artery available for distal reconstruction may be the distal peroneal or distal anterior tibial artery.

A bypass is then performed from the proximal popliteal artery cephalad to the aneurysm as well as distal anastomosis to a target artery which is patent. It is important to perform completion arteriography. We have used intraoperative TPA (4 mg) in the target artery as a one-time dose in patients with a limited runoff. Following bypass, there is potential of reperfusion injury often requiring fasciotomy.

Results

Kropman et al. reported the results from 8 prospective studies and 25 retrospective studies including 895 patients diagnosed with PAA presenting with acute ischemia from 1990 to 2008; the mortality rate after surgical repair was 3.2% [2]. Thrombolysis before surgery did not result in a significant reduction in the number of amputations compared with surgery (thrombectomy or bypass) alone. The mean primary patency rates of the bypasses at 1, 3, and 5 years were 79%, 77%, and 74%, respectively, in the thrombolysis group and 71% ($P = 0.026$), 54% ($P = 0.164$), and 45% ($P = 0.249$), respectively, in the thrombectomy group. From a Swedish vascular registry, 717 primary operations for PAAs in 571 patients were registered prospectively from 1987 to 2002, with 235 legs presenting with acute ischemia [3]. Immediate surgery was performed on 135 legs including intraoperative thrombolysis in 32 cases (immediate surgery group). Preoperative thrombolysis was performed on 100 legs, followed by acute cases (less than 24 h) on 41 legs; elective surgery was performed on 59 legs (delayed surgery group). The delayed surgery group had smaller PAA (27 versus 37, $P < 0.001$) and was younger (67 versus 72 years, $P < 0.001$) [3]. Runoff was worse in the delayed surgery group than in the immediate surgery group ($P < 0.001$) and improved in 87% after thrombolysis. The amputation rate was 27% in immediate surgery group and 7% in the delayed surgery group ($P < 0.0001$). The immediate surgery group required fasciotomy in 30% compared to 11% in delayed surgery group ($P = 0.0001$) [3].

Case 1

A 68-year-old man presented to the emergency room with a sudden onset of pain in the left lower extremity associated with paresthesia with limited ability to move his ankle and toes and with absent leg DP and PT Doppler flow (Rutherford Grade II B). CTA showed abrupt occlusion of the left popliteal artery above the knee and with a filling defect behind the knee; there was 1.7 cm dilation of the left popliteal artery without discernable contrast (Figs. 14.1 and 14.2a, b). There was a faint visualization of the left posterior tibial artery in the distal calf and ankle.

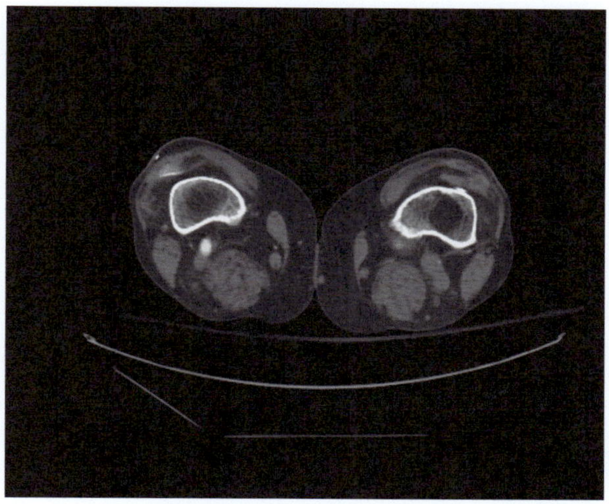

Fig. 14.1 CTA showing the thrombosed left popliteal aneurysm (axial image)

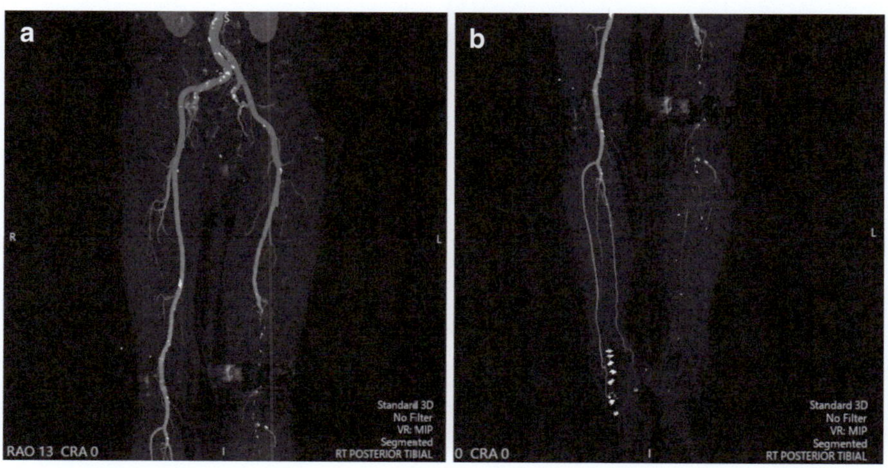

Fig. 14.2 (**a**) CTA showing the thrombosed left popliteal artery aneurysm. (**b**) CTA showing the thrombosed left popliteal aneurysm with poor runoff

He was emergently taken to the OR and underwent thrombectomy of the left popliteal artery using left femoral arteriotomy with a Fogarty balloon catheter. There was absent Doppler flow in the popliteal artery, posterior tibial artery, and dorsalis pedis artery in the foot. The left posterior tibial artery at the ankle was exposed using in situ bypass the left femoral artery to the distal post tibial artery achieved a satisfactory outcome. Duplex imaging of the graft 3 months postoperatively showed patient bypass but with stenosis at the distal anastomosis. CT angiography showed patent left femoral-distal posterior tibial in situ bypass with mild stenosis just distal to the distal anastomosis (Fig. 14.3a–c).

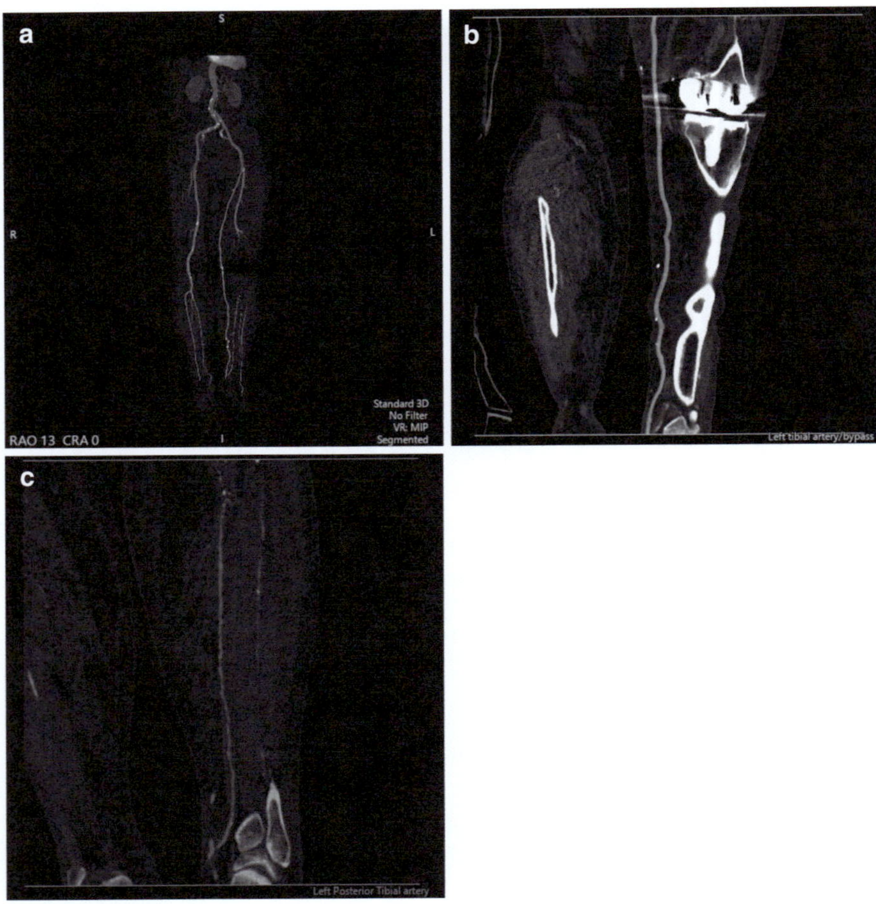

Fig. 14.3 (**a**) Postoperative CTA showing the occlusion of the left popliteal artery with a patent left patent femoral-distal-posterior tibial bypass. (**b**) Postoperative CTA showing in situ bypass in the lower thigh and below the knee. (**c**) Postoperative CTA showing mild stenosis beyond distal anastomosis

Case 2

A 64-year-old man presented to the emergency room with sudden onset of pain and paresthesia in the right lower extremity with loss of motor function in the distal right lower extremity. CTA showed a small AAA and bilateral large popliteal aneurysms with thrombosis of the right popliteal aneurysm (Fig. 14.4). Because of limb-threatening ischemia, the patient underwent exposure of the large left popliteal aneurysm using a medial approach. Popliteal artery distal to the popliteal aneurysm was opened longitudinally, and a passage of a No. 3 Fogarty catheter did not retrieve any thrombi with absent retrograde flow. The DP artery at the ankle was exposed, and arteriotomy in the DP revealed a small amount of back bleeding. The patient underwent proximal popliteal to the DP bypass using the translocated right great saphenous vein with completion arteriogram (Fig. 14.5). As reperfusion resulted in a marked bulging of the calf muscles, a fasciotomy was performed. The patient subsequently developed interval ischemic necrosis of the medial calf (skin and muscle) and had multiple debridements and skin grafts (Fig. 14.6). The patient developed thrombosis of the graft and underwent a thrombectomy of the graft, and the graft was rerouted and brought through the interosseous membrane and anastomosed to the DP artery with interposition of a short segment of non-reversed GSV. Despite patency of the bypass graft, the patient required above-knee amputation of the leg because of extensive necrosis of the skin and muscles of the calf. Patient died 4 years later due to persistent congestive heart failure.

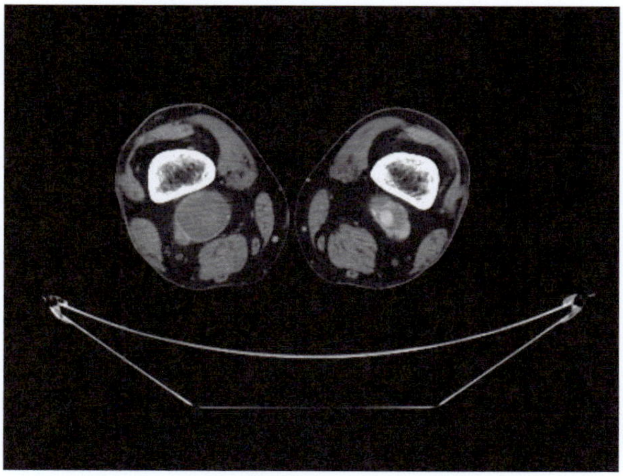

Fig. 14.4 Bilateral large popliteal aneurysms with thrombosis of the right popliteal aneurysm

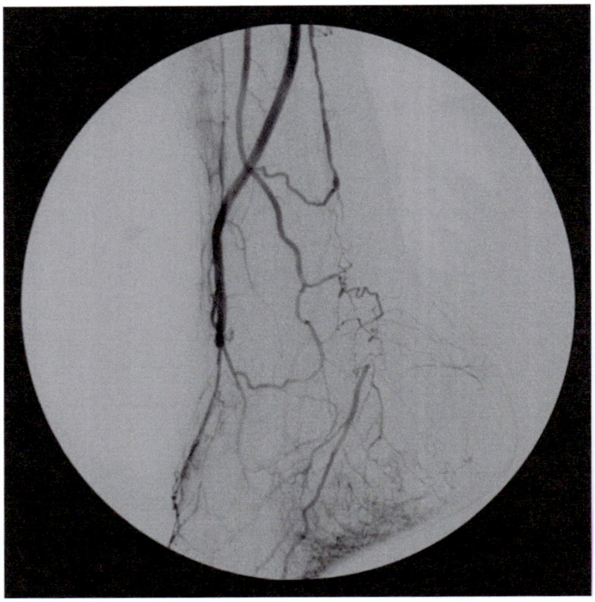

Fig. 14.5 Completion of arteriogram showing vein bypass to the dorsalis pedis artery following open repair of the thrombosed popliteal aneurysm

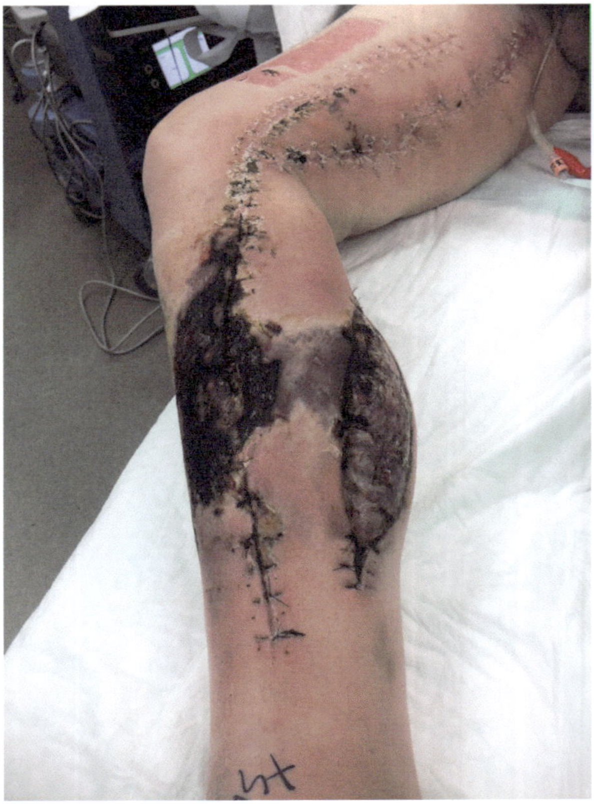

Fig. 14.6 Photograph of right medial calf showing ischemic necrosis

Invited Commentary

Krish Soundarajan, MD, MBA

Acute thrombosis of popliteal artery aneurysm is a dreaded limb-threatening vascular emergency. Limb loss up to 60% has been reported, but more recently with use of intraoperative thrombolysis, the incident has reduced considerably to about 14–17%.

When presented with nonviable limb, patients are best managed with early amputation. However, when patients present with impending ischemia, they need to be emergently addressed, more often by open surgery rather than endovascular therapy.

Fluoroscopic-assisted embolectomy can be a valuable adjunct if the intraoperative angiogram shows multiple outflow vessel occlusions. I prefer an over-the-wire, triple lumen Fogarty balloon catheter that not only serves well for a guided atraumatic embolectomy, but also to check individual outflow vessels without needing to reenter the tibioperoneal arteries.

When performing open surgery, in terms of distal anastomosis, an end to side would be a better configuration when it is performed above the tibioperoneal outflow and when more than one vessel is at least partially patent. However, when there is a single vessel outflow, an end to end is likely to serve well, depending on the exposure and accessibility during surgery.

With increasing endovascular interventions of aortic aneurysms and screening for popliteal aneurysms becoming more common, it is likely that popliteal aneurysms will be electively managed, and hence, acute thrombosis of popliteal aneurysms is likely to become much less prevalent.

References

1. Rutherford RB. Clinical staging of acute limb ischemia as the basis for choice of revascularization method: when and how to intervene. Semin Vasc Surg. 2009;22(1):5–9.
2. Kropman RH, Schrijver AM, Kelder JC, Moll FL, de Vries JP. Clinical outcome of acute leg ischaemia due to thrombosed popliteal artery aneurysm: systematic review of 895 cases. Eur J Vasc Endovasc Surg. 2010;39(4):452–7.
3. Ravn H, Björck M. Popliteal artery aneurysm with acute ischemia in 229 patients. Outcome after thrombolytic and surgical therapy. Eur J Vasc Endovasc Surg. 2007;33(6):690–5.

Ruptured Popliteal Aneurysm

15

Most patients with popliteal artery aneurysms (PAAs) are diagnosed on account of an incidental mass in the back of the knee, or fortuitously during a duplex imaging series of the lower extremity performed for an unrelated diagnosis. Some patients with PAA present with symptoms of lower extremity ischemia or ischemia due to thrombosis of the popliteal aneurysm, as described in Chap. 14. Rupture of the popliteal aneurysm is uncommon and has been reported in only 2–5% of patients with PAA [1, 2]. Cervin et al. reported 45 patients presenting with ruptured PAA based on a Swedish vascular registry (1987–2012), which represented 2.5% of all patients who underwent repair of PAA [1]. In their series, patients presenting with rupture were on anticoagulants in 50% of the cases. Patients presenting with rupture were 8 years older than those patients presenting with intact popliteal artery aneurysms; out of 45 cases, 42 had open repair and 3 had endovascular repair. Thirty-day outcomes showed patency of the reconstruction in 35 patients and amputation in 4 out of 45 patients within 1 week of surgery, with a 1-year survival rate of 60%.

Most patients present with contained rupture in the lower right thigh or knee area as a painful pulsatile mass. Free rupture of PAA is uncommon. Patients should undergo emergency CTA of the abdominal aorta and lower extremities and be taken to a hybrid OR following resuscitation. A groin cut-down is performed, and CFA/SFA is exposed, and an antegrade arteriogram is performed. If there is extreme tortuosity of the artery proximal and distal to the aneurysm, open repair is preferable. In patients with a relatively straight course of the SFA and distal popliteal artery, proximal and distal to PAA, an endovascular approach is preferable. In our experience, in elderly patients with multiple comorbidities, endovascular repair in the presence of one-vessel runoff is still the preferred method. Results of endovascular repair in the presence of poor runoff (one-vessel) are inferior to those with two- or three-vessel runoff.

Most popliteal artery aneurysms present as an asymptomatic pulsatile mass behind the knee. The results of treatment for asymptomatic popliteal aneurysm with open repair as well as endovascular repair are satisfactory. A primary patency rate

S. S. Hans, *Contemporary Management of Lower Extremity Aneurysmal Disease*,
https://doi.org/10.1007/978-3-032-00159-7_15

of 86.5% has been reported [3]. Among symptomatic patients, results are better in those with symptoms of intermittent claudication than those with acute ischemia or rupture of the aneurysm. A rupture of popliteal aneurysm is relatively uncommon and occurs in only 3–7% of patients with popliteal aneurysm, but the number of reported cases is quite small; therefore, short-term and long-term results in this group remain ill defined [4]. Patients with contained rupture present with a painful pulsatile mass behind the knee with subcutaneous ecchymosis associated with severe pain and tenderness in the knee area. The risk of amputation is much higher in patients with a rupture or acute ischemia than in patients presenting chronic ischemia. Other symptoms of popliteal aneurysm rupture include deep venous thrombosis and peroneal nerve palsy.

Though acute rupture of a popliteal artery aneurysm is rare and initial clinical presentation can be nonspecific, this possibility must be entertained when dealing with older male patients presenting with a pulsatile mass associated with pain in the lower medial thigh or posterior aspect of the knee. Such patients should undergo duplex ultrasound of the knee area and/or CTA to rule out popliteal aneurysm rupture. It is extremely uncommon to have a free rupture from popliteal artery aneurysm because patients often have a contained rupture and are usually hemodynamically stable. Endovascular repair with a covered stent graft is possible in only a small group of patients in which the popliteal artery proximal and distal to the aneurysm has a relatively straight course. In the presence of extreme tortuosity, endovascular repair may be difficult to perform. An open repair with interposition of PTFE graft though saphenous vein graft is preferable.

Cervin et al. reported 45 patients with ruptured popliteal artery aneurysm from the Swedish vascular registry (1987–2012). The proportion of ruptured popliteal aneurysm was 2.5% of all patients who were operated with popliteal artery aneurysm in their registry [5]. Patients presenting with a rupture of the popliteal aneurysm were on anticoagulants in about 50% of the cases. Out of 45 patients, 42 had an open repair and 3 had an endovascular repair. Those with ruptured popliteal aneurysms were 8 years older than those treated with intact popliteal artery aneurysms [5]. Thirty-day outcome showed patency of reconstruction in 35 out of 39 and amputation in 4 out of 45 occurrences with a 1-year survival rate of 60% [5]. Bani-Hani et al. treated a ruptured infected popliteal artery aneurysm in an 85-year-old male with angioplasty of distal popliteal and tibial peroneal trunk and posterior tibial artery in order to improve distal outflow prior to deployment of two overlapping GORE®VIABAHN® Endoprosthesis stent grafts (7 × 15 and 8 × 15) [6]. The patient developed infected hematoma in the lower thigh necessitating incision and drainage and was started on rifampicin and daptomycin as cultures grew *Staphylococcus aureus* and group G streptococcus [6].

Case 1

A 70-year-old male with history of chronic obstructive pulmonary disease secondary to bronchial asthma and remote nicotine abuse had been in an extended care facility for 9 months. He had been ambulating with significant pain in the right knee and right calf when he was brought to the emergency room of the hospital and was found to have a painful pulsatile mass in the lower thigh (Fig. 15.1). CTA of the right lower extremity revealed a contained rupture of the right popliteal aneurysm with marked tortuosity of the distal superficial femoral artery and popliteal artery junction (Fig. 15.2).

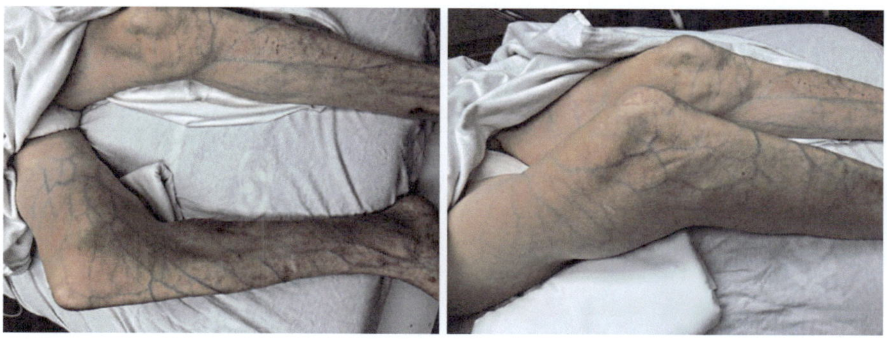

Fig. 15.1 (**a** and **b**) Large swelling on the medial and posterior aspect of the right lower thigh

Fig. 15.2 CTA showing a large popliteal aneurysm

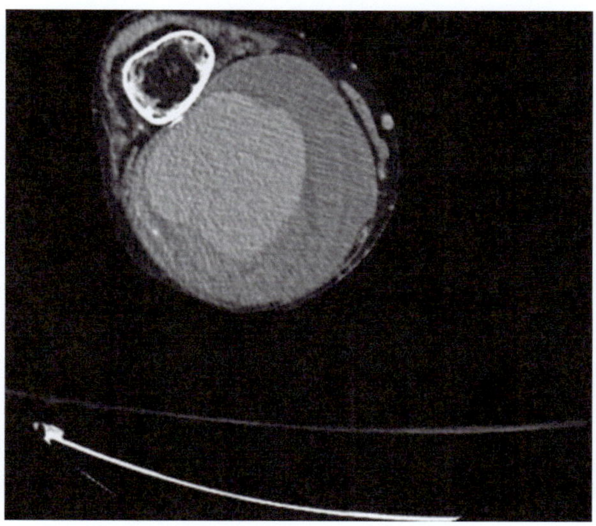

The patient was taken to the hybrid operating room for possible endovascular repair/possible open repair. Using an antegrade approach with a micropuncture technique, a 5F sheath was advanced to obtain an arteriogram, which showed marked tortuosity of the distal right superficial femoral artery and a large giant popliteal aneurysm with eccentric origin of the distal popliteal artery above the knee (Fig. 15.3). Multiple attempts via a long 6F sheath and together with a Kumpe catheter and an angled soft GLIDEWIRE (0.035 mm) were made to negotiate the popliteal artery distal to the aneurysm, but we could not advance the wire into the popliteal artery and its outflow tract. The sheath was removed, and incision was made from the middle of the thigh to the upper calf with division of the tendon of the adductor magnus, and exposing the junction of the distal superficial femoral and popliteal artery, a silastic vessel loop was passed. Another incision was made in the upper calf, the medial head of the gastrocnemius and the tendons of pes anserinus were divided, and a silastic vessel loop was passed around the distal popliteal artery. The patient was given 5000 units of heparin via anesthesia. The aneurysm was very large with a hematoma in its wall (Fig. 15.4), and there was also a hematoma around

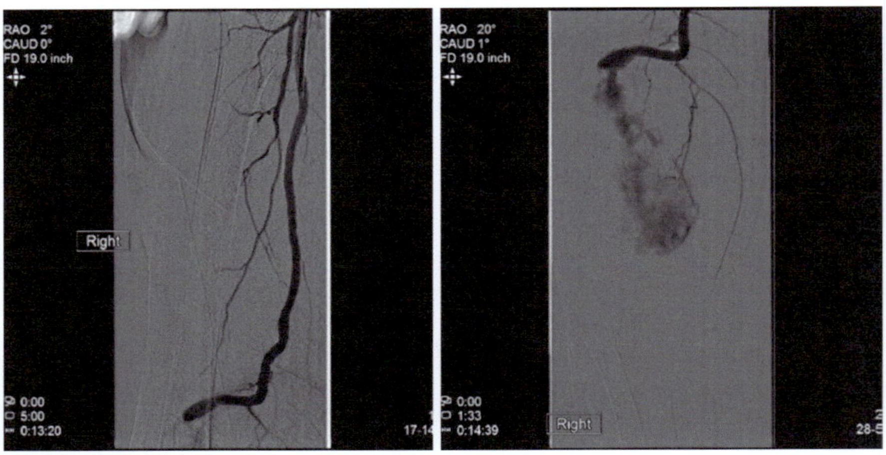

Fig. 15.3 Arteriography (in the operating room) showing a large aneurysm with thrombus and extreme tortuosity of the distal superficial femoral artery

Fig. 15.4 Operative picture showing a large popliteal aneurysm with hematoma in the outer wall

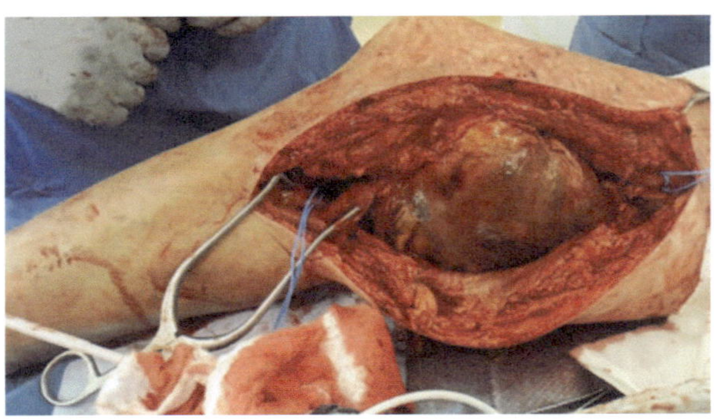

the wall of the aneurysm which was indicative of contained leak. Vascular clamps were applied proximal and distal to the aneurysm, and the aneurysm was opened (Fig. 15.5). The anterior wall of the aneurysm was removed, as well as all the laminated thrombus. The distal superficial femoral artery and popliteal artery were mobilized, and an 8 mm PTFE PROPATEN® graft (W.L. Gore, Newark, DE) was selected for proximal anastomosis to be performed end-to-end with 5-0 cardiovascular polypropylene running suture. Distally, the popliteal artery was mobilized and divided distally to the aneurysm making a T-shaped opening in the popliteal artery. Distal anastomosis was performed using the same suture (Fig. 15.6). There was satisfactory back bleeding from the distal popliteal artery, and distal anastomosis was performed end-to-end as well. The patient had excellent Doppler flow in the posterior tibial and dorsalis pedis artery. The wound was closed in layers, and a Jackson-Pratt drain was inserted in the popliteal fossa and removed after 48 h (Fig. 15.7). In this patient, the greater saphenous vein was inadequate, and the

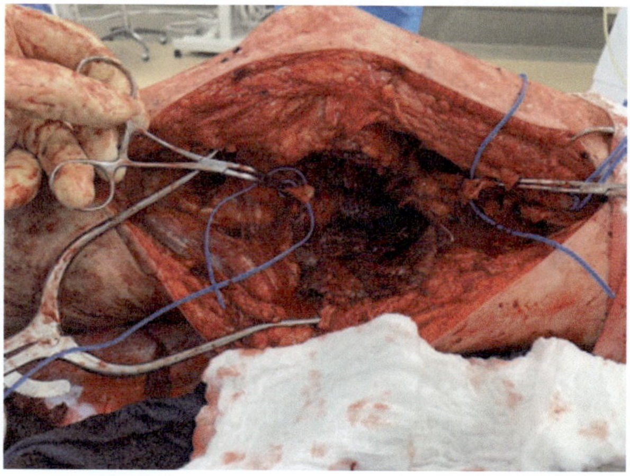

Fig. 15.5 Resection of the aneurysm and divided proximal and distal end of popliteal artery with vascular clamp

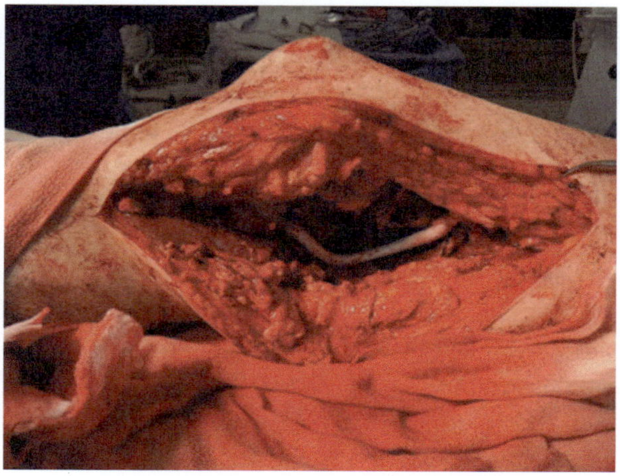

Fig. 15.6 Interposition of an 8 mm PTFE graft

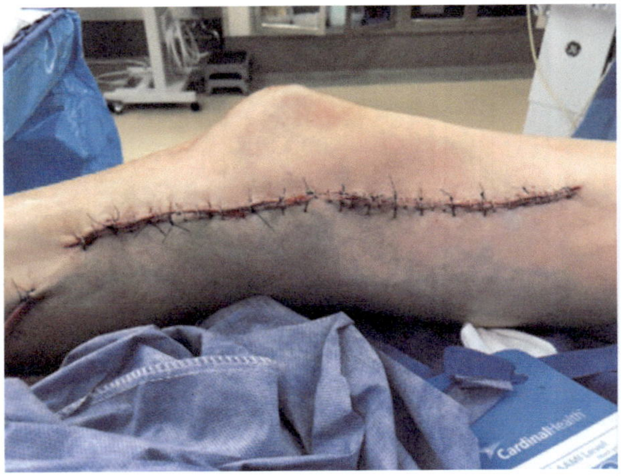

Fig. 15.7 Skin closure

patient's general condition was suboptimal; therefore, a PTFE graft was preferred. The patient was seen for a follow-up 9 months later and found to be in satisfactory condition and ambulating with the help of a cane.

Case 2

An 84-year-old male presented to the emergency room with pain and swelling of the left lower thigh of 10-day duration. The patient's symptoms developed during his exercise routine when he felt a "pop" in his left lower thigh on April 19, 2007. Duplex examination showed a large pseudoaneurysm in the distal left superficial femoral artery. Medical comorbidities included coronary artery disease with prior coronary artery bypass graft (CABG) and chronic renal failure (creatinine 1.9 mg/dL), and the patient was on warfarin. He received 4 units of fresh frozen plasma for an INR of 4.5 and was then taken to the hybrid operating room.

A 5 F sheath was inserted in the right femoral artery percutaneously, and aortic bifurcation was visualized by a small amount of contrast injection via right femoral sheath, which showed aneurysmal dilatation of the distal abdominal aorta in both common iliac arteries. The left common iliac artery, left external iliac artery, and left femoral artery were selected using an Omniflush catheter, and the arteriogram showed diffuse dilatation of the left superficial femoral artery. In addition, there was evidence of extravasation of the contrast of the distal thigh from a large distal superficial femoral artery/proximal popliteal aneurysm (Fig. 15.8).

Using GLIDEWIRE® (Terumo Interventional Systems, Somerset, NJ) and Kumpe catheter (Cook Medical, Bloomington, IN), we were able to advance the catheter just proximal to the site of the rupture and obtain an arteriogram which showed that the aneurysm extended to the distal popliteal artery and was lined with a small amount of thrombus. In this patient, the left greater saphenous vein had been harvested from the left lower extremity for a remote CABG, and because of

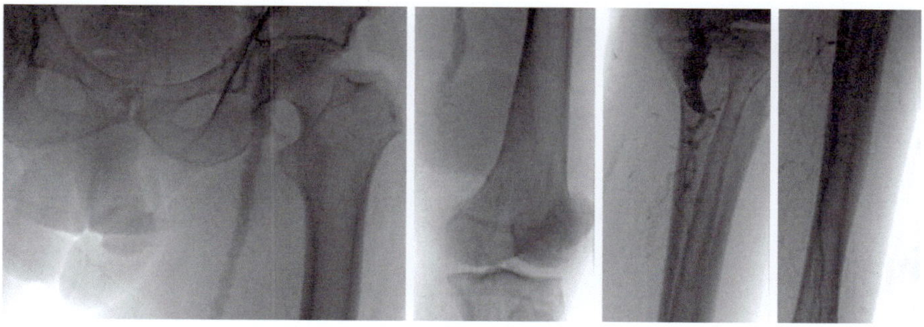

Fig. 15.8 The left superficial femoral artery, popliteal artery, and large popliteal aneurysm with runoff with peroneal artery

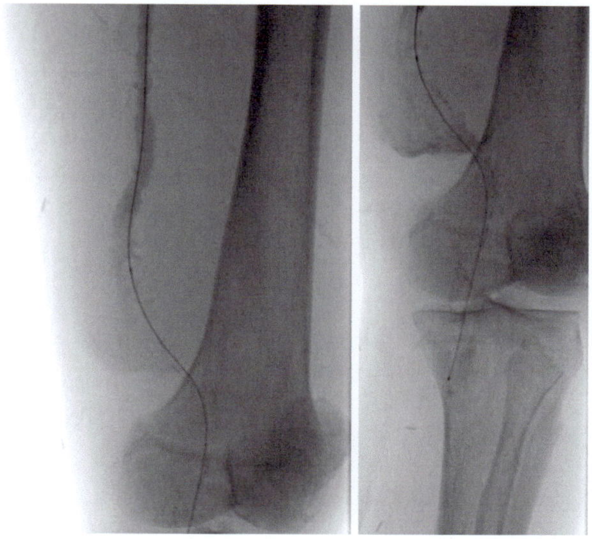

Fig. 15.9 Guidewire access into the distal popliteal artery

significant medical comorbidities, it was decided to do an endovascular repair. The smaller 5F sheath was exchanged for a 10 F long arrow sheath, which was placed in the left mid-superficial artery. An exchange length of 0.035/260 cm long GLIDEWIRE® was advanced from the ruptured segment into the distal popliteal artery (Fig. 15.9). Three Fluency® stents (Bard Peripheral Vascular, Tempe, AZ), measuring 10 × 60, 10 × 60, and 10 × 40 with an overlapping 5–6 mm segment, were deployed with complete exclusion of the ruptured aneurysm (Fig. 15.10). A follow-up duplex study showed patent stent graft with complete exclusion of the aneurysm. A FemoStop™ (Abbot, Chicago, IL) was applied to the right groin. The patient had a Doppler arterial signal in the posterior tibial and dorsalis pedis artery because the runoff in this patient was only with the peroneal artery, which was occluded in its proximal 3–4 cm length. Both posterior tibial and interior tibial

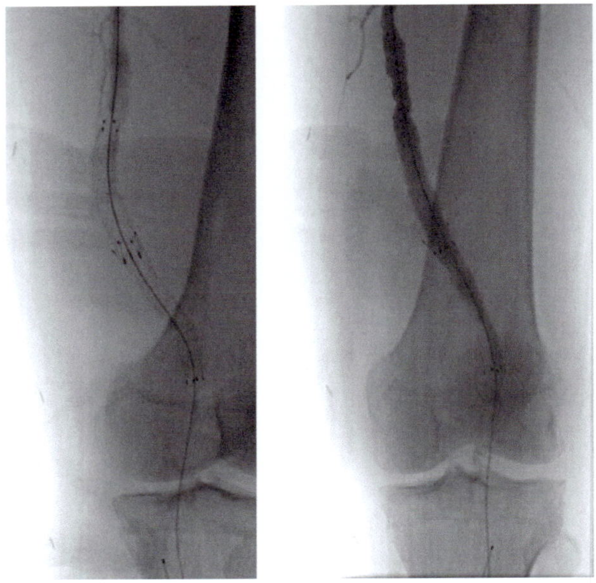

Fig. 15.10 Deployment of three Fluency® stents and successful exclusion of a large popliteal aneurysm

arteries were occluded. The patient was readmitted on May 3, 2007, with a right groin necrotic wound at the site of the entry of 10 F sheath. The wound was debrided, and the patient was started on IV antibiotics. He was discharged on May 6, 2007 and died 2 years later from an unrelated cause.

Invited Commentary

Paul Bove, MD, FACS

The authors crystalize the complexity of the entity of ruptured popliteal artery aneurysm.

In the elective setting, the most common of peripheral aneurysms, the popliteal artery aneurysm, has unique characteristics with respect to presentation, identification, and treatment. It is not infrequent in occurrence and commonly bilateral with a male preponderance. The diagnosis by primary care physicians is often difficult to detect on physical exam and more commonly found on unrelated diagnostic testing such as an incidental finding on venous duplex ultrasonography or when evaluating arterial insufficiency on lower extremity arterial testing with arterial duplex ultrasonography. PAA can be less commonly identified in other radiographic studies such as CT, MRI, or conventional radiographs. The asymptomatic patient with PAA is the most common presentation, with chronic or acute limb ischemia being the second most common. As in ruptured PAA, open and endovascular repair is often performed sometimes with the adjunct of thrombolysis in the case of acute limb ischemia to identify or enhance runoff, often impacting outcome.

The chapter and following case presentations by the authors detail the complexities not only in treating patients with PAA but the enhanced complexity of those with ruptured PAA. As noted, when compared to the elective PAA patients, ruptured patients often are more elderly, with increased comorbidities, and, not infrequently, on anticoagulant medications. In addition to the rupture, the patients may have concomitant acute or chronic ischemia. In addition, venous or nerve compression is more frequent, and the potential for compartment syndrome exists. All of which may require decompression even if an endovascular approach is utilized for revascularization. The cases presented clearly demonstrate the unique procedural challenges of patients with this complex diagnosis and should be commended. The nuances to the treatment algorithms are well described in the chapter and demonstrated by the cases presented and should assist future vascular providers when presented with this clinical situation.

References

1. Cervin A, Ravn H, Björck M. Ruptured popliteal artery aneurysm. Br J Surg. 2018;105(13):1753–8.
2. Sie RB, Dawson I, van Baalen JM, Schultze Kool LJ, van Bockel JH. Ruptured popliteal artery aneurysm. An insidious complication. Eur J Vasc Endovasc Surg. 1997;13(5):432–8.
3. Pulli R, Dorigo W, Troisi N, et al. Surgical management of popliteal artery aneurysm: which factors affect outcome? J Vasc Surg. 2006;43:481–7.
4. Sie RB, Dawson I, VanBaalan JM, et al. Ruptured popliteal artery aneurysm: and insidious complication. Eur J Vasc Endovasc Surg. 1997;13:432–8.
5. Cervin A, Ravn H, Bjorck M, et al. Ruptured popliteal aneurysm. Br J Surg. 2012;105:1752–8.
6. Bani-Hani MG, Elnahas L, Plant GR, Ward A, et al. Endovascular management of ruptured infected popliteal artery aneurysm. J Vasc Surg. 2012;55:532–4.

16 Infrapopliteal Artery Aneurysm

Aneurysms involving the infrapopliteal arteries are rare occurrence. The vast majority are pseudoaneurysms and mycotic aneurysms involving the tibioperoneal trunk and its branches in association with bacterial endocarditis. Many true aneurysms of the infrapopliteal arteries are associated with concomitant systemic diseases such as vasculitis or Ehlers-Danlos syndrome [1–4]. A careful history-taking, physical examination, and serological tests for vasculitis and collagen diseases should be performed to rule out connective tissue disorders.

Most patients are diagnosed by coincidence during diagnostic imaging for peripheral arterial disease [1–4]. Patients may present with cramping pain due to swelling of the leg caused by venous obstruction. CTA or MRA is often diagnostic in such cases (Fig. 16.1). Arteriography provides useful information in planning treatment, but is not necessary; CTA images can provide the required information (proximal artery, outflow) for planning the arterial reconstruction. Rupture is rare, but thrombosis and peripheral embolization can be limb threatening. Resection with interposition view (GSV) is preferable for small asymptomatic aneurysms involving the infrapopliteal arteries, which can be observed with serial duplex imaging. In patients with concurrent popliteal artery and infrapopliteal aneurysms, the following options were described by Aziz et al. (Fig. 16.1) [3].

1. Endovascular treatment of popliteal and tibioperoneal trunk aneurysms. This will require multiple stent grafts depending on the distance from the distal SFA and the site of the aneurysm in the tibioperoneal trunk with increased risk of thrombotic complication.
2. Open treatment of both popliteal and tibioperoneal trunks with an autologous GSV is the best option, provided adequate length is available.
3. Endovascular repair of the popliteal artery and bypass for tibioperoneal trunk aneurysm.
4. Surgical bypass for popliteal aneurysm and stent graft placement for tibioperoneal trunk aneurysm (Fig. 16.2a, b). The decision to select the best management

S. S. Hans, *Contemporary Management of Lower Extremity Aneurysmal Disease*,
https://doi.org/10.1007/978-3-032-00159-7_16

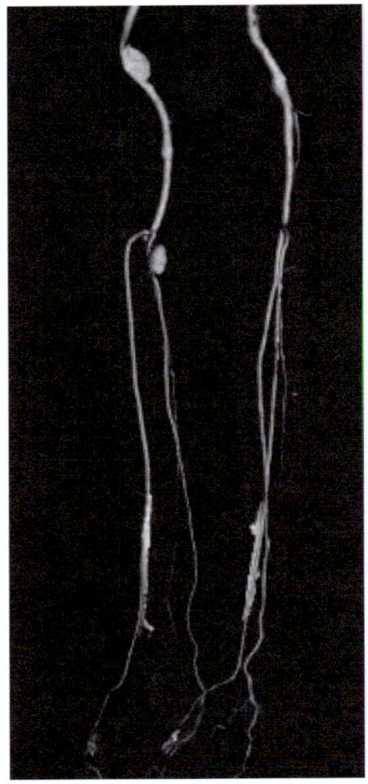

Fig. 16.1 CTA of the lower extremities showing a 1.8 cm aneurysm of the right tibioperoneal trunk in addition to a popliteal artery aneurysm. (Courtesy of Dr. Faisal Aziz)

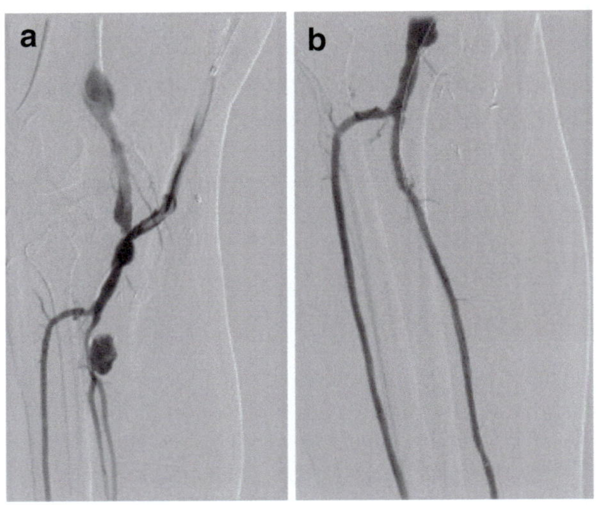

Fig. 16.2 (**a**) Arteriogram showing the hybrid approach—after bypassing the popliteal artery aneurysm, a balloon-expandable stent graft is placed in the tibioperoneal trunk. (Courtesy of Dr. Faisal Aziz). (**b**) Arteriogram showing the distal runoff of the posterior tibial artery and anterior tibial artery with sacrifice of the peroneal artery. (Courtesy of Dr. Faisal Aziz)

option depends on the required length of the stent graft for popliteal aneurysm, exclusion availability of adequate length and quality of GSV, and patient's general medical condition.

Mycotic Aneurysms of the Tibioperoneal Trunks

In the past, most mycotic aneurysms were the result of arterial embolization due to bacterial endocarditis. Since the widespread use of newer antibiotics, the incidence of mycotic aneurysms has decreased significantly in the presence of valvular heart disease. There has been an increase in the incidence of peripheral mycotic aneurysms due to intravenous drug abuse. Large bilateral tibioperoneal trunk aneurysms were reported in a patient 6 weeks after mitral valve replacement (MVR) due to *Streptococcus viridans* endocarditis.

The management of popliteal and infrapopliteal aneurysms can be challenging and depends on the adequacy of collateral circulation. If the collateral circulation is adequate, ligation and excision of the mycotic aneurysm with a concomitant antibiotic and/or a consultation with an infectious disease specialist should be undertaken. Most infection disease specialists recommend 6 weeks of antibiotic therapy.

If collateral circulation is inadequate, revascularization with autologous vein bypass should be performed. Synthetic grafts should be avoided. The source of the mycotic embolism such as vegetations in the heart valve should be treated by a cardiothoracic surgeon.

References

1. Mönig SP, Walter M, Sorgatz S, Erasmi H. True infrapopliteal artery aneurysms: report of two cases and literature review. J Vasc Surg. 1996;24(2):276–8.
2. Katz SG, Kohl RD, Razack N. Bilateral infrapopliteal artery aneurysms. Ann Vasc Surg. 1992;6(2):168–70.
3. Aziz F, Pooshpas P. Hybrid repair of concurrent popliteal artery and tibioperoneal trunk aneurysms. J Vasc Surg. 2019;69(5):1596–8.
4. Murashita T, Yasuda K, Takigami T, Sakuma M, Matsui Y, Sasaki S, Shiiya N. Mycotic aneurysm of the bilateral tibioperoneal trunks associated with bacterial endocarditis: a case report. Int Angiol. 1997;16(3):176–9.

Popliteal Venous Aneurysm

17

Popliteal vein aneurysms are a rare condition that necessitates repair because of the associated high risk of venous thrombosis and of pulmonary embolism. Several mechanisms have been proposed for the pathogenesis of venous aneurysm ranging from reflux and venous hypertension, inflammation, infection, congenital vein wall weakness, mechanical trauma, and localized degenerative change with loss in the focal normal connective tissue components in the vein wall is the most accepted theory. The endophlebohypertrophy and endophlebosclerosis are the main histological features [1]. The focal structural changes of the venous wall may be related to the increased expression of select matrix metalloproteinases. The structural changes in the aneurysmal segment include a single irregular lumen, diminished smooth muscle components, increased fibrous tissue, fragmented elastin fibers, and sparse infiltration with inflammatory cells [1]. Venous aneurysms rarely rupture.

Preoperative diagnostic studies include duplex venous imaging and magnetic venous resonance venography (Figs. 17.1 and 17.2). A preoperative venogram is not routinely required.

S. S. Hans, *Contemporary Management of Lower Extremity Aneurysmal Disease*,
https://doi.org/10.1007/978-3-032-00159-7_17

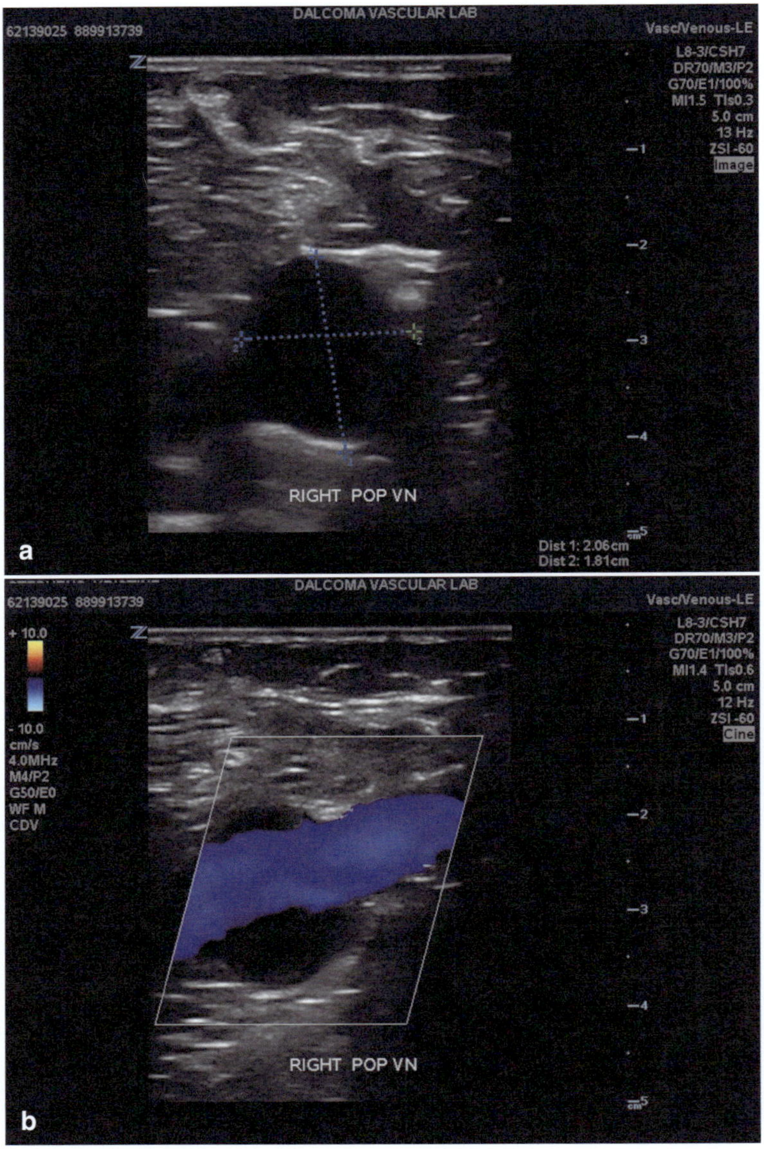

Fig. 17.1 (**a**) Duplex ultrasound of the popliteal vein aneurysm. (**b**) Color duplex ultrasound showing the longitudinal view of the popliteal aneurysm with partial thrombus

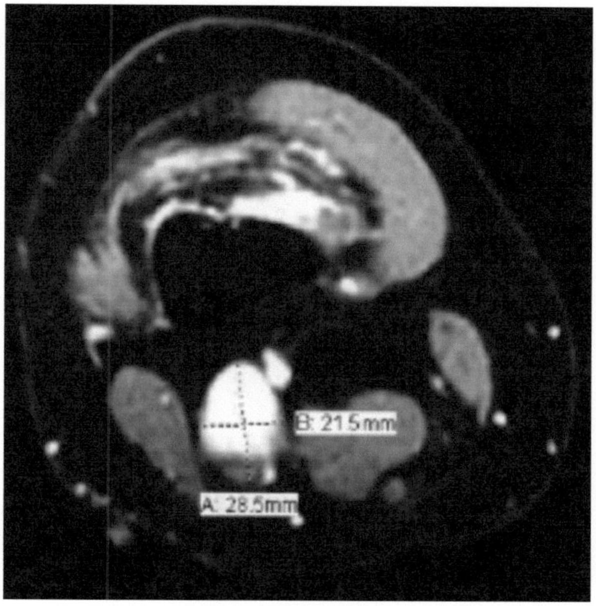

Fig. 17.2 Magnetic resonance venography of the popliteal vein aneurysm. The image shown is an axial T1 fast spoiled gradient-echo FS postcontrast magnetic resonance imaging

Operative Management

Several options of operative repair have been reported. If there is redundant length of the vein proximal and distal to the venous aneurysm, resection with end-to-end anastomosis of the proximal and distal segments of vein without tension is a suitable option. If additional length of the vein is required to avoid any tension at the anastomosis resection followed by an interposition graft, harvesting of the graft from the GSV or femoral vein can be performed. Generally, a vein with diameter of 2 cm, as seen on duplex imaging in an upright position with turbulent flow, is considered an indication for repair.

Tangential aneurysmectomy and lateral venorrhaphy are also considered suitable options (Fig. 17.3). In the presence of thrombosis, open thrombectomy before plication is performed. Patients undergo duplex venous ultrasound in preoperative holding room for identification of popliteal venous aneurysm and are assessed for thrombus. Posterior approach for exposure is preferable, and general anesthesia is induced in supine position before turning the patient. A "lazy" S-shaped incision is made over the posterior aspect of the knee, overlying the popliteal space horizontally with superior extension of the incision medially and the inferior extension laterally. The incision is deepened, and subcutaneous tissues are divided with electrocautery. During the exposure, sural nerve and the small saphenous vein are identified and retracted gently. The posterior tibial nerve is identified and gently dissected free. Interoperative duplex is performed after venous aneurysm is exposed with inflow and outflow vein diameter to help determine the specific luminal diameter required following plication. The proximal and distal popliteal vein is encircled

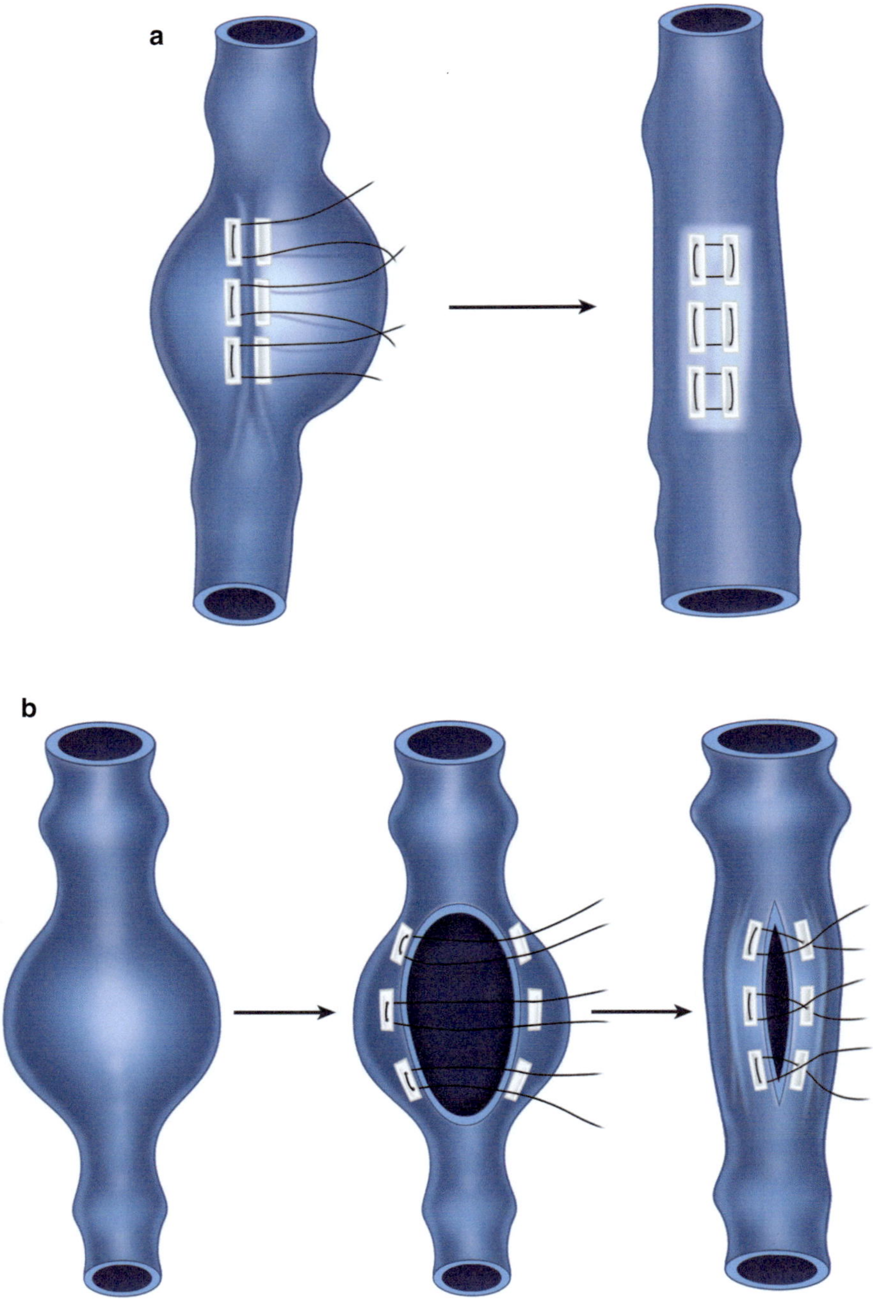

Fig. 17.3 (**a**) Popliteal vein aneurysm plication. Note the pledgeted sutures. (**b**) Popliteal vein aneurysm excision of the redundant vein tissue (dark with cross-checks) with closure. Note the pledgeted sutures

with a silastic loop; systemic heparization is not necessary in the absence of the thrombosis in the aneurysm. Plication of the aneurysm is performed with interrupted horizontal mattress sutures using 6.0″ Cu polypropylene (ETHICON, Cincinatti, OH) with felt pledgets [1] (Fig. 17.3).

If a thrombus is present in the popliteal venous aneurysm, the patient is given intravenous heparin to keep the target activated clotting time (ACT) between 250 and 300 seconds. After obtaining proximal and distal control, a longitudinal venotomy is performed and extended to an approximate length, and thrombus is removed, and closure in pledgets is performed as previously described [1, 2].

After plication is performed, intraoperative duplex ultrasound assesses the venous flow through the repair, and if the diameter of the repair vein closely approximates that of the native vessel, the wound is closed in layers. Postoperative early ambulation is started with the use of elastic compression stockings. If thrombus was present in the aneurysm at the time of repair, a 3-month course of anticoagulants should be considered [1].

Results and Major Complications

There is paucity of data pertaining to popliteal venous aneurysm repair. Sessa et al. reported 25 patients undergoing repair of popliteal venous aneurysm with no report of recurrent PE following repair [1, 3]. They reported a complication rate of 20%, which included transient peroneal nerve palsy, wound infection, hematuria, and postoperative thrombosis of the repaired segment.

Invited Commentary

Sashi Inkollu, MD

Popliteal venous aneurysms (PVA) are the most common venous aneurysms but are still quite rare. Management is dependent on the size, and repair is indicated when >2 cm due to the risk of deep venous thrombosis and pulmonary embolism. Lifelong anticoagulation is a viable option for those who are not operative candidates. The chapter describes the management of PVAs including operative technique in detail. I personally prefer a venorrhaphy or aneurysmorrhaphy. The risk of thrombosis is always higher on the venous side of the circulation as compared to the arteries due to the slower flow velocities, and hence, prosthetic must be avoided whenever feasible.

The amount of vein to resect or plicate can be tricky to determine once the venous aneurysm is open. One way is to use the mathematical formula:

$$C = \pi d$$

The circumference of the vein can be measured from edge to edge, and resection can be guided by the number obtained using intended final diameter (Figs. 17.4 and 17.5).

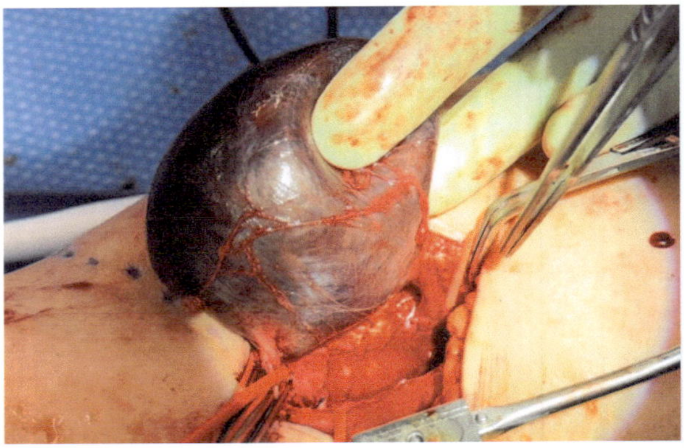

Fig. 17.4 Popliteal vein aneurysm dissected and mobilized out of the fossa with proximal and distal control

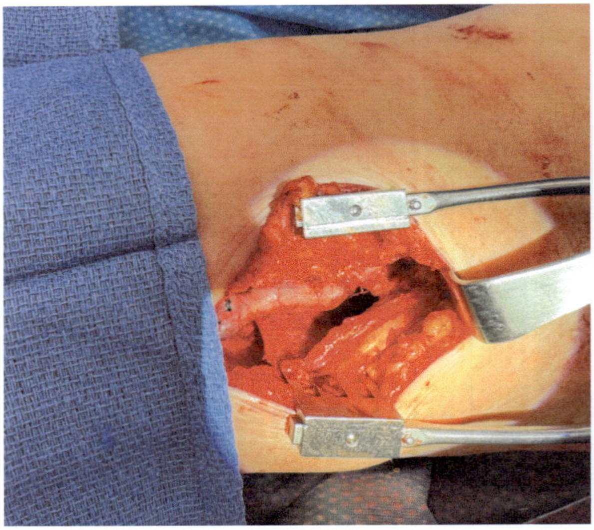

Fig. 17.5 Image after repair with venorrhaphy

References

1. Robinson S, Downing T, Coleman D, Williams DM, Wakefield TM. Endovascular/Open central and peripheral venous reconstruction. In: Hans SS, Shepard AD, Weaver MR, Bove P, editors. Endovascular and open vascular reconstruction: a practical approach. CRC Press; 2017. p. 391–402.
2. Noppeney T, Kopp R, Pfister K, Schierling W, Noppeney J, Cucuruz B. Treatment of popliteal vein aneurysms. J Vasc Surg Venous Lymphat Disord. 2019;7(4):535–42.
3. Sessa C, Nicolini P, Perrin M, Farah I, Magne JL, Guidicelli H. Management of symptomatic and asymptomatic popliteal venous aneurysms: a retrospective analysis of 25 patients and review of the literature. J Vasc Surg. 2000;32(5):902–12.

Management of Femoral Artery Pseudoaneurysm with AV Fistula

18

Most femoral artery venous (AV) fistulas are acquired due to the penetrating trauma during diagnostic or interventional cardiovascular procedures involving femoral artery and femoral vein access. Acquired femoral AV fistula may also be the result of penetrating knife wounds or a gunshot injury. Associated pseudoaneurysms with acquired fistula are uncommon. During percutaneous access, lateral or medial needle deviation can lead to a simultaneous puncture of the artery and the accompanying vein; once there is a simultaneous puncture and the needle is withdrawn, the communication between the artery and the vein may not seal, resulting in the formation of arteriovenous fistula; occasionally, there is an accompanying pseudoaneurysm from the puncture site in the artery. The large common femoral artery and vein fistulas can result in hemodynamic changes due to short circuiting of the blood from the high-resistance arterial circulation to the low-resistant venous channel, resulting in significant increase in the venous volume as well as venous pressure. This results in the decrease of the peripheral vascular resistance, increasing stroke volume and heart rate with possible increase in cardiac output. High-flow arteriovenous fistula may result in diminished blood flow to the extremity and, in the presence of preexisting lower extremity arterial occlusive disease, worsening of ischemic symptoms [1].

Risk factors for iatrogenic arteriovenous fistula include increased body mass index, advanced age, hypertension, and female gender. Patients with punctures inferior to the common femoral artery (CFA) or profunda femoris artery (PFA) punctures, patients with multiple punctures, and patients on anticoagulation are at increased risk for iatrogenic femoral AV fistula. Low groin punctures may result in a simultaneous puncture of the SFA or deep femoral artery because this may result in puncture of the profunda vein. Ultrasound-guided access is more likely to result in the single-wall puncture of the common femoral artery.

S. S. Hans, *Contemporary Management of Lower Extremity Aneurysmal Disease*,
https://doi.org/10.1007/978-3-032-00159-7_18

Clinical Presentation and Diagnostic Studies

Following combined arterial and venous punctures, AV fistulas that appear are usually clinically asymptomatic except in patients with associated pseudoaneurysm [1, 2]. A tender pulsatile mass may be palpable with an audible bruit, and there may be ecchymosis at the puncture site in the groin. A small number of arteriovenous fistulas (up to 2%) may resolve spontaneously, but there may be a new onset of symptoms of intermittent claudication. Long-standing femoral AV fistulas may result in edema of the lower extremity due to venous hypertension or aneurysmal changes in the wall of the artery; and in large fistulas, high-output cardiac failure may result or may make the heart failure more probable in a patient with compensated heart failure. Congestive heart failure is more likely to occur in long-standing untreated femoral arteriovenous fistula.

Color duplex ultrasound is the initial diagnostic modality of choice for suspected patients with femoral arteriovenous fistula. Color duplex ultrasound offers high-frequency, low-resistance continuous flow with elevated diastolic velocities through the pulse cycle. The exact location of a fistulous opening may not be clearly determined by CTA or MRA diagnosis, but there is simultaneous filling of the external iliac artery and the external iliac vein (Fig. 18.1a, b). Catheter-based digital subtraction angiography (DSA) is the diagnostic modality of choice as the fistula's communication is better delineated with rapid opacification of the deep vein (Fig. 18.2).

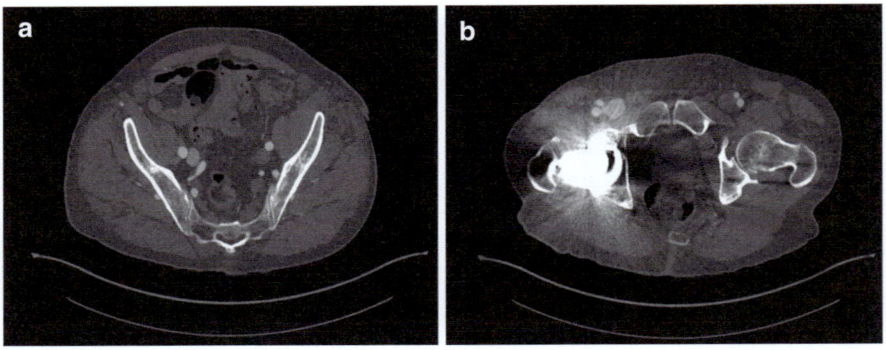

Fig. 18.1 (**a**) CTA showing the simultaneous filling of the right external iliac artery and the vein. (**b**) CTA showing the simultaneous filling of the right common femoral artery and the vein

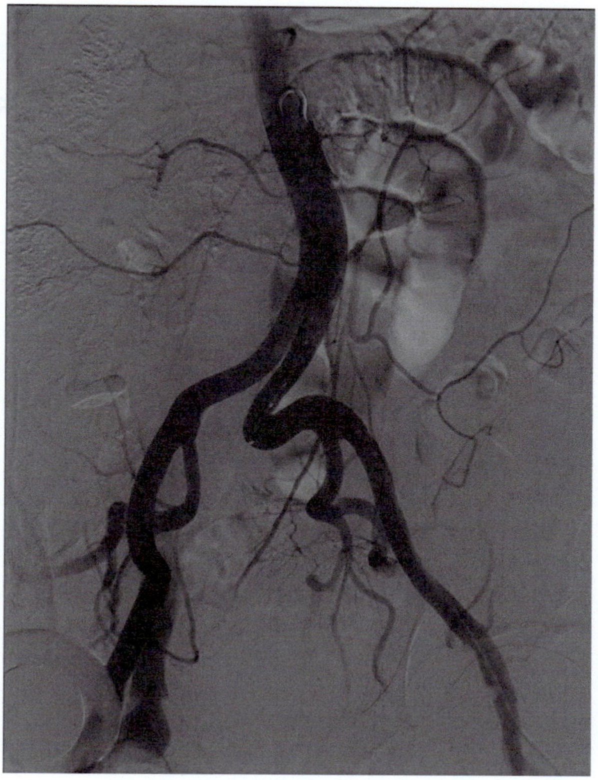

Fig. 18.2 Arteriography showing the simultaneous filling of the right femoral and external iliac vein due to femoral arterial venous fistula

Management

Repair is indicated:

1. In patients with significant redirection of blood into venous system resulting in distal limb ischemia
2. Significant venous hypertension in the lower extremity
3. Large AV fistula following gunshot or stab injury
4. Iatrogenic AVFs without spontaneous resolution as most AV fistulas will usually resolve within 1 year of occurrence

Endovascular Repair

Placement of a covered stent with or without coil embolization should be considered in high-risk patients, with hostile groin (prior surgery with scar tissue). Covered stent deployment in the common femoral artery should be avoided due to the potential of deformation and stent fracture. Iatrogenic fistulas that originate from the proximal SFA just distal to CFA bifurcation or from deep PFA are more suitable for covered stent placement in high-risk patients; however, there is increased risk of stent thrombosis in such patients. In high-risk patients with appropriate imaging of the fistulous connecting channel, percutaneous deployment of detachable coils or a N-butyl-cyanoacrylate embolic agent is an occasional option. In patients with delayed diagnosis of iatrogenic AV fistulas, a hybrid approach with open repair and subsequent coil embolization may have to be considered.

Open Surgical Repair

Open surgical repair is usually the most satisfactory option for the repair of femoral arterial-venous fistula under general anesthesia and by the use of a hockey-stick incision in the groin extending to the upper thigh. Because of venous hypertension and friable vessels, there is a potential for excessive bleeding; therefore, arrangements for possible blood transfusion should be made. The femoral sheath is opened, and proximal and distal control of the common femoral artery and superficial and deep femoral artery should be obtained depending on the site of arterial-venous communication. The proximal and distal control of the vein is not usually necessary and may result in excessive bleeding from a tear of a small tributary of the femoral vein. Manual compression with a Kittner sponge proximally and distally from the site of AV fistula helps control venous blood loss. If a fistula connection cannot be ascertained, operative duplex imaging should be obtained. The defect in the artery and the vein should be closed with a polypropylene suture (5″0′ or 6″0′). In long-standing fistulas, the dissection of the artery can be difficult, and dissection should be done in the periadventitial plane.

Complications of Repair

1. Excessive bleeding
2. Surgical site infection

Case Example

An 82-year-old man presented a palpable mass in the right groin. The patient had a history of electrophysiology procedure performed 6 months earlier involving right femoral venous access. A duplex study revealed pseudoaneurysm involving the right proximal superficial femoral artery. CT angiography showed a pseudoaneurysm associated with the proximal right superficial femoral artery and an AV fistula with a communication between the proximal segment of the superficial femoral artery to the femoral vein. The patient was scheduled for the repair of the fistula and pseudoaneurysm.

The left common femoral artery was punctured under ultrasound guidance with micropuncture technique, and a microsheath was advanced. Through the microsheath, a J-wire was advanced, and then a 5-French sheath was also advanced. Through the

5-French, an Omniflush catheter was placed in the abdominal aorta, and an abdominal aortogram was obtained, which showed significant tortuosity of the left common iliac artery in the middle segment of almost 90 degrees as well as tortuosity of the infrarenal abdominal aorta. With repeated attempts and a number of catheters used including internal mammary artery catheter (Glidecath and initially Omniflush catheter), we were able to advance the wire into the right common femoral artery; however, the catheter could not be tracked into the distal external iliac artery. As a 6F 45-cm-long pinnacle sheath could not be advanced, the proximal balloon occlusion of the femoral artery was abandoned. A hockey-stick incision was made just above the upper thigh. Dissection was somewhat challenging because of the chronic inflammatory changes surrounding the fistula. The veins were very prominent; the shelving edge of the inguinal ligament was exposed, and under that, the common femoral artery was exposed; it was larger in caliber than average, and a vessel loop was passed in the common femoral artery. The dissection was done around the pseudoaneurysm with exposure of the proximal superficial femoral artery just inferior to the pseudoaneurysm. The deep femoral artery could not be visualized. The common femoral vein was separated from the common femoral artery as well as the proximal superficial femoral vein, and the origin of the profunda vein was visible. The patient was given 6000 units of heparin. A double-vessel silastic loop was passed around the proximal common femoral artery and proximal superficial femoral artery, and vascular clamps were applied proximally and distally.

A pseudoaneurysm was opened, and a large amount of thrombus were removed since there was an opening in the anterior wall of the artery, which was contributing to the pseudoaneurysm. The pseudoaneurysm was closed with interrupted 5-0 cardiovascular horizontal mattress sutures. The dissection proceeded to the junction of the profunda femoral vein, and with the common femoral vein, significant venous bleeding from an opening in the profunda femoris vein was encountered and was carefully controlled using DeBakey forceps and a 4-0 cardiovascular Prolene suture. There was a tear in the posterior wall of the proximal superficial femoral artery, which was closed with horizontal mattress sutures of 5-0 cardiovascular Prolene suture. There was a through-and-through opening in the proximal superficial femoral artery probably caused by the puncture for the electrophysiology procedure. The patient had excellent pulse distal to the repair of the femoral artery. Irrigation was performed with heparinized saline. A 10 mm Jackson drain was inserted through a separate stab incision, and a subcutaneous suture was applied with interrupted 2-0 Vicryl, 3-0 Vicryl; the skin was sutured with 3-0 nylon and staples. Patient was seen 6 months after the repair with satisfactory closure of arteriovenous fistula.

Invited Commentary

Peter Henke, MD

Pseudoaneurysms (PSA) are a common vascular iatrogenic injury that vascular surgeons routinely see and treat. Those with an associated arteriovenous fistula (AVF) are less common. Overall, femoral PSA have likely decreased due to the use of radial artery access for cardiac and peripheral catheterization, but many procedures are still done through the groin due to size and anatomy in which the catheter-based approaches are used to treat. A traumatic AVF is usually caused by the needle traversing both the vein and artery as noted in the chapter. It is amazing that these AVF stay patent, even if the initial sheath size is not that large. It is rare in our experience for these to be particularly symptomatic. Most of the time, they are discovered incidentally when a duplex is ordered to evaluate a pseudoaneurysm.

Treatment of most femoral pseudoaneurysms is with duplex-guided thrombin injection. However, this technique may be hazardous if an AVF is present, as the thrombin injection could enter the venous system, causing deep vein thrombosis. Many times, the pseudoaneurysm may resolve on its own, and the AVF remains. For these patients, it has been our practice to usually follow them expectantly. The number of AVF that have required open resection and division is probably 1 or 2 per decade, based on anecdotal experience from our institution.

Patients may have small AV fistulas for years, which rarely cause any type of limb symptoms or high-output cardiac congestive heart failure. As noted in the chapter, those that are large or related to some other types of traumatic injury do merit a repair in most cases. These can also occur in the setting of patients with a connective tissue disorder, such as Ehlers-Danlos type IV. If the patient has the connection between the superficial femoral artery and the branch of the vein or the vein itself, a covered stent is a minimally invasive option as noted. Open surgical repair is often harder than expected because the AVF are often quite difficult to find, despite a good duplex image. Nonetheless, this nicely written and detailed chapter for this situation highlights the essential techniques and indications for repair of the pseudoaneurysm with an AV fistula.

More broadly, the PSA with or without an AVF further supports direct ultrasound-guided micropuncture technique for all arterial procedures, rather than based on feel or experience alone.

References

1. Stone P. Acquired arteriovenous fistula of the lower extremity. In: Connor RF, editor. UpToDate. Wolters Kluwer. Accessed 1 July 2024.
2. Nagpal K, Ahmed K, Cuschieri R. Diagnosis and management of acute traumatic arteriovenous fistula. Int J Angiol. 2008;17(4):214–6.

Popliteal Artery and Venous Pseudoaneurysm with Arteriovenous Fistula

19

Popliteal arteriovenous fistulas occur because of penetrating trauma (gunshot or stab wounds) [1–4]. Cases of popliteal artery pseudoaneurysm and AV fistula have been reported following arthroscopy. Stab injury in the proximal calf or inadvertent laceration of the genicular branches of popliteal artery during the placement of a trocar for arthroscopy can cause popliteal artery venous fistulas or popliteal artery pseudoaneurysms. During meniscectomy, the neurovascular bundle may be injured because of its close proximity to the posterior horn of the meniscus. Popliteal pseudoaneurysm and arteriovenous fistula following acupuncture has also been reported. Spontaneous popliteal AV fistulas caused by popliteal aneurysms in patients with Marfan syndrome, human immunodeficiency virus, and arteritis have also been reported. The diagnosis is initially suspected by the location of the penetrating injury, associated history of arterial bleeding, and, in chronic cases, symptoms of venous hypertension with or without venous ulceration, arterial steal, and occasionally high-output heart failure. Delay in the diagnosis of popliteal pseudoaneurysms and arteriovenous fistula is relatively common. Following penetrating trauma, delay of up to 2 years in the diagnosis of pseudoaneurysms and AV fistula has been reported.

Duplex ultrasound, CTA, and MRA are diagnostic tools that help in planning treatment options. Catheter-based arteriography is required in most cases to delineate the communication.

Management options include open surgical repair, endovascular repair, and hybrid repair. Endovascular and hybrid repair is preferable in chronic popliteal artery arteriovenous fistula with multiple arterialized segments. In the presence of associated pseudoaneurysm and popliteal arteriovenous fistulas without significant arterialized varicosities, open repair is preferrable [1, 2].

For open repair, direct ligation of the communication takes place; then, arterial repair is performed. If primary repair is not feasible without undue tension, a short interposition graft, preferably using GSV, should be performed. An endovascular option includes deployment of a covered stent and coil embolization or deployment of a vascular plug. The advantages of endograft repair include lower morbidity and

S. S. Hans, *Contemporary Management of Lower Extremity Aneurysmal Disease*,
https://doi.org/10.1007/978-3-032-00159-7_19

mortality, a shorter length of stay, and a shorter recovery time. Disadvantages include risk of stent thrombosis and fracture [2].

Case Example

A 73-year-old woman with a 6-month history of chronic knee pain was found to have a medial meniscus tear and underwent arthroscopy with a partial posterior horn medial meniscectomy. Three days postoperatively, she developed increased calf swelling and posterior knee and leg pain and was unable to bear weight on the affected extremity. On examination, a palpable mass was noted in the popliteal fossa without a thrill and with palpable distal dorsalis pedis and posterior tibial pulses. The patient underwent a duplex ultrasound to evaluate for deep venous thrombosis (DVT) and was found instead to have a vascularized mass in the popliteal fossa and without evidence of DVT.

Computed tomography angiography (CTA) of the lower extremity demonstrated simultaneous opacification of both the femoral artery and the femoral vein in the arterial phase (Fig. 19.1a, b). Within the popliteal fossa, a large vascular structure was seen consistent with a pseudoaneurysm measuring 3.7 cm in its greatest antero-posterior diameter. There was also noted an AV fistula between the popliteal artery and the vein. Arteriography demonstrated simultaneous filling of the popliteal artery and vein and delayed filling of a large venous pseudoaneurysm (Fig. 19.2a, b). The AV fistula was again revealed just below the pseudoaneurysm although its exact origin was difficult to delineate. A high takeoff of the anterior tibial artery was visualized.

Through a posterior popliteal fossa approach, the patient underwent an operative ligation of the arteriovenous fistula and venous pseudoaneurysm. Bleeding from the venous pseudoaneurysm was controlled by lateral venography using monofilament

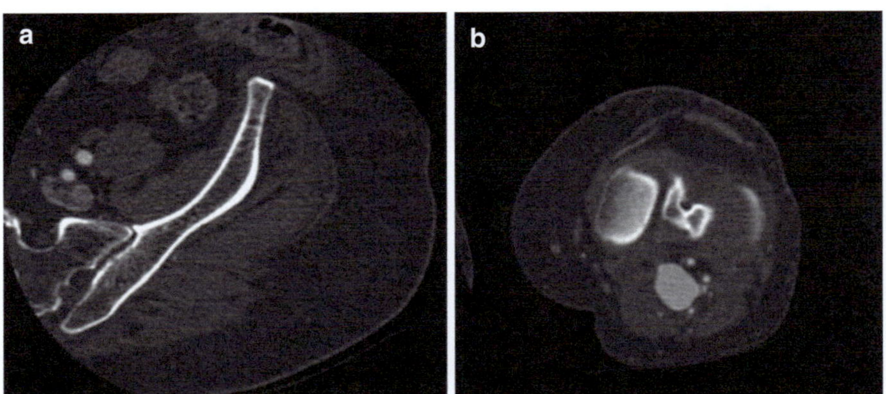

Fig. 19.1 (**a**) CTA demonstrating simultaneous two-vessel opacification (external iliac artery and vein) at the level of the pelvis which extended into the popliteal fossa. (**b**) Demonstrates the large pseudoaneurysm during arterial phase in the popliteal fossa

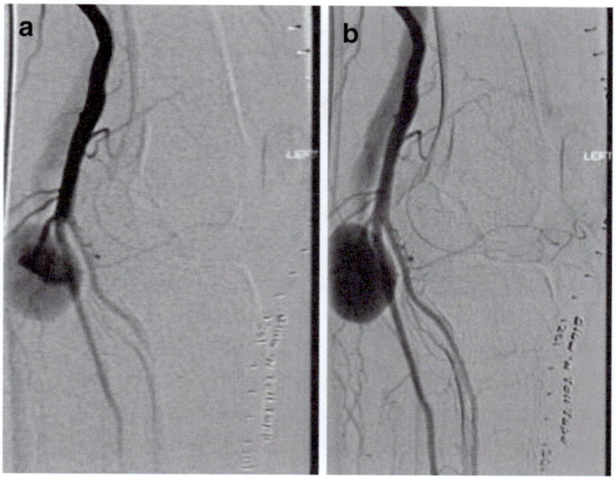

Fig. 19.2 (**a**) An angiographic image demonstrating AP views in the arterial phase and with two-vessel opacification and delayed filling of the pseudoaneurysm. (**b**) Lateral projections demonstrate the arteriovenous fistula communication to the venous pseudoaneurysm

polypropylene suture (Ethicon, Cincinnati, OH). A large intramuscular hematoma was evacuated from the medial head of the gastrocnemius muscle. The patient tolerated the procedure well and was discharged home 5 days later.

On postoperative day 12, the patient returned to the emergency department with increased swelling and pain. At this time, duplex venous imaging demonstrated a posterior tibial vein thrombus and nonvascularized mass of 4.0 cm consistent with residual hematoma. The patient was considered a high risk for progression of DVT and therefore treated with 3 months of anticoagulation with Coumadin. She returned for follow-up duplex at that time with no further evidence of DVT or hematoma and regained full function and weight-bearing capacity of the left leg.

Several known complications of knee arthroscopy including bleeding, infection, and deep venous thrombosis have been reported [3]. Less common complications include arterial or vascular injury, nerve injury, and injury to the articular cartilage. Delayed presentation of arterial pseudoaneurysms and arteriovenous fistula following meniscectomy has been reported, but venous pseudoaneurysm and AV fistula arising from the genicular artery have not been reported from our review of the literature [3].

The most plausible explanation for this complication was the inadvertent laceration of the genicular arteries during the placement of the medial arthroscopic trocar. In this patient, an arteriovenous fistula formed between the genicular artery and the vein with pulsatile flow into the aneurysmal popliteal vein with resulting contained rupture and formation of a pseudoaneurysm. Alternatively, during manipulation and external rotation of the knee, the neurovascular bundle approximates the attachment of the posterior horn of the meniscus and may be injured during the meniscectomy [3]. This patient had a preexisting popliteal venous aneurysm, which ruptured due to high pressure caused by the arteriovenous fistula resulting in pseudoaneurysm formation. The venous aneurysm ruptured into a closed space creating pseudoaneurysm (PSA). The possibility of a vascular injury must be considered in all patients with new onset of pain and evidence of popliteal fossa fullness or mass post-arthroscopy. In a previously published case of a venous pseudoaneurysm of the popliteal vein, the PSA was repaired with polypropylene, but the arterial injury required a short segment bypass graft [3]. In our patient, the bypass graft was not required, as the arterial injury was to the genicular arteries sparing significant trauma to the popliteal artery.

Treatment strategies vary depending on the type and location of an injury. Increasing popularity of endovascular control of post-arthroscopy arterial pseudoaneurysms has been reported using covered stents in the popliteal region with good results [3]; however, this case highlights the importance of getting lateral views during arteriography to confirm the origin of the pseudoaneurysm before planning intervention. If in doubt, an open repair and direct ligation should be performed with or without short segment bypass depending on the degree of arterial trauma.

Persistent pain and swelling of the lower extremity following knee arthroscopy should raise suspicion about vascular complications such as popliteal vein thrombosis or arterial pseudoaneurysm, and prompt duplex ultrasound imaging of the knee should be obtained [4].

Invited Commentary

Tamer N. Boules, MD

This chapter highlights the primary causes of popliteal pseudoaneurysm and arteriovenous fistula—penetrating trauma. Although traumatic injury to the popliteal artery can occur as a result of stabbing or be gun-related, iatrogenic penetrating injuries related to orthopedic procedures are well described and can involve the popliteal artery proper or its geniculate branches, as the authors have eloquently described. Most of these iatrogenic injuries are identified acutely, as they are associated with expanding hematomas within confined compartments, significant edema, as well as coexisting ischemic complications from arterial thrombosis.

However, other iatrogenic causes also need to be mentioned as popliteal approaches have become common for arterial and venous endovascular procedures. Direct injury from through-and-through needle or sheath access is possible and has been reported. Indeed, with the increasing use of postoperative anticoagulation and dual antiplatelet agents, iatrogenic popliteal arteriovenous fistulas and pseudoaneurysms are less likely to close or thrombose spontaneously, analogous to their more frequent common femoral counterparts. Finally, although less common in the modern era where CT angiographic evaluation is widely used, delayed presentation of popliteal arteriovenous fistula can occur even years after injury if not noted immediately after penetrating/blunt trauma where "hard" signs of arterial trauma are not acutely evident and further imaging with CT or duplex are not performed.

In terms of management, as the authors have highlighted, the priority is to define the location of the injury and differentiate direct popliteal arteriovenous injury from branch injury. Although simple coil embolization of injured geniculate arterial branches is straightforward, open drainage of associated large hematomas to decompress tense compartments may be required. If the popliteal artery is directly involved, less invasive procedures using covered stent grafts can be employed, but their long-term patency is questionable especially in younger patients who frequently have smaller normal vessels prone to spasm and thrombosis. Although stent grafts can be used as a temporizing treatment strategy in the unstable patient, open repair frequently via a posterior approach, with possible greater saphenous vein interposition arterial reconstruction, and direct repair of the vein are necessary in the majority of patients, as the authors have stated.

In the setting of a delayed presentation, where symptoms of venous hypertension or steal are well established, catheter-based angiography may be necessary to define the exact location of the abnormal communications between artery and vein, especially when the fistula is large or high-flow, making localization by CT angiography alone challenging. Although stent-grafting can also be considered in the chronic setting when a direct popliteal arteriovenous fistula is identified, this may not be ideal, as there may be significant size discrepancy with a large hypertrophied artery just proximal to the communication and a small "decompressed" artery just distal to it. In general, appropriately "auto-tapering" self-expanding stent-grafts are not widely available, and infolding of an oversized straight stent-graft within a small artery carries higher risks of future thrombosis. Finally, when approaching complex arteriovenous fistulas using open techniques, especially in the setting of traumatic anatomic distortion and engorged venous branches, use of tourniquets or other endovascular techniques for proximal/distal control should be considered as adjuncts to minimizing blood loss.

Although rapid access and widespread application of CT angiography has expedited the diagnosis and treatment of traumatic popliteal arteriovenous fistulas and pseudoaneurysms, future efforts focus on prevention and early detection of iatrogenic injuries. Maintaining a high index of suspicion guided by mechanism is critical when evaluating bleeding or injury involving popliteal structures, even when external signs and symptoms are subtle, and should result in accelerated imaging with duplex or CTA. Ultrasound guidance has become the standard when popliteal venous or arterial access is necessary during vascular procedures, and is being used similarly at some centers during arthroscopic surgery to assist port placement and avoid neurovascular injury.

References

1. Soumer K, Benomrane S, Derbel B, et al. Popliteal pseudoaneurysm and arteriovenous fistula after acupuncture. J Mal Vasc. 2015;40(1):58–62.
2. Ying A, Al-Asady R, Vicaretti M. Endovascular treatment of a large iatrogenic popliteal arteriovenous fistula. J Vasc Surg Cases Innov Tech. 2020;6(1):129–32.
3. Hans SS. Popliteal venous pseudoaneurysm and associated arteriovenous fistula following knee arthroscopy. In: Hans SS, editor. Challenging arterial reconstructions: 100 clinical cases. Cham: Springer; 2020. p. 265–7.
4. Alserr AH, Antonopoulos CN, Papapetrou A, et al. Endovascular repair of popliteal artery pseudoaneurysm with arteriovenous fistula after knee arthroscopy: case report and literature review. Vasc Endovasc Surg. 2014;48(2):166–70.

Lower Extremity Fasciotomy 20

Compartment syndrome (CS) of the lower extremity is the result of increased pressure in a limited space compromising the circulation, which results in ischemia of the muscles and nerves occupying that space. Unless promptly treated, this increased compartment pressure will ultimately result in loss of nerve and muscle function causing permanent deformity of the extremity or, at worst, limb loss [1–4]. Prompt diagnosis and management of the condition is mandatory to preserve muscle function and prevent amputation of the extremity [1–4]. Two common causes of compartment syndrome encountered by vascular surgeons are reperfusion following delayed establishment of arterial flow caused by thromboembolic disease or following arterial reconstruction for an acute thrombosis of the popliteal artery aneurysm. A more common cause of compartment syndrome occurs following arterial vascular trauma caused by reperfusion injury following revascularization or direct soft tissue injury or hemorrhage within the fascial compartments. Other causes of compartment syndrome include phlegmasia cerulea dolens and revascularization following combined arterial and venous injury. Risk factors for the development of compartment syndrome are as follows: greater than 6 hours of ischemia time, younger age, hypotension, paucity of collaterals, and location of the arterial occlusion. The incidence is higher following combined popliteal, arterial, and venous injuries.

Compartment pressure in the lower extremity is normally 10–12 mm Hg. It has been suggested that a compartment pressure of 30 mm Hg should be used as a threshold for the diagnosis of compartment syndrome [4, 5]. Diagnosis of compartment syndrome is most often made based on clinical criteria. Pain out of proportion to an injury or severe pain in the calf after revascularization out of proportion to the expected incisional pain is suggestive of compartment syndrome. Pain is worsened by a passive stretch such as dorsiflexion of the foot, sensorimotor deficits, palpable swelling, and tenseness of the lower leg. Kleckner et al. reported the strongest predictors of fasciotomy wherein patients with extremity arterial trauma injury showed an ischemia time exceeding 2.5 h, Rutherford category of ischemia of II a, a higher location (popliteal artery segment) and type (transection and occlusion), male

S. S. Hans, *Contemporary Management of Lower Extremity Aneurysmal Disease*,
https://doi.org/10.1007/978-3-032-00159-7_20

gender, and the mechanism of injury [3]. The liberal use of prophylactic fasciotomy substantially improves the historically poor rate of limb salvage and function following popliteal vascular trauma [3].

Fasciotomy is the definitive treatment including complete incision and decompression of the skin and investing fascia of each of the four lower leg compartments.

Four Lower Leg Compartments (Fig. 20.1)

1. Superficial posterior compartments containing the gastrocnemius and soleus muscles
2. Lateral compartment containing the peroneal muscles and the superficial peroneal nerve
3. Anterior compartment containing the anterior tibial vessel nerves and the dorsiflexors of the foot
4. Deep posterior compartment containing the posterior tibial and peroneal vessels and the tibial nerve and muscles including flexor hallucis longus, flexor digitorum longus, tibialis posterior, and popliteus

Two longitudinal incisions in the lower leg—medial and lateral—are used to expose the compartment. Fibulectomy is not necessary to decompress the lateral compartment [5].

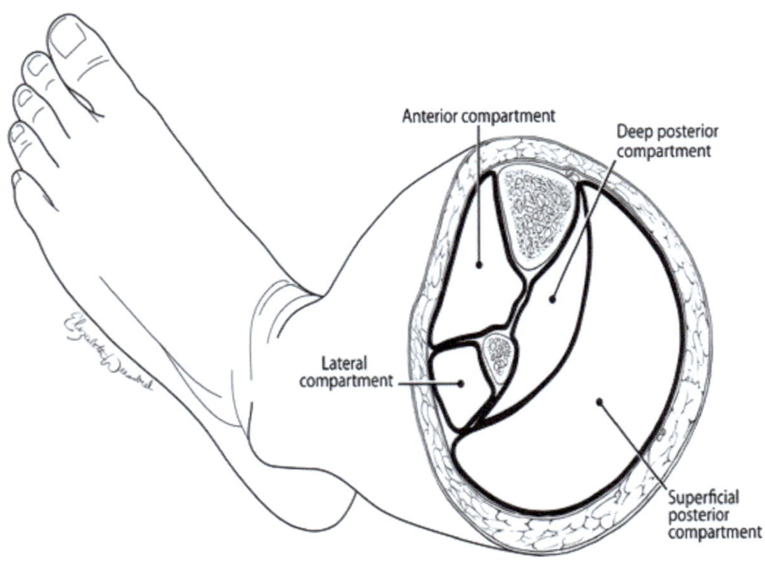

Fig. 20.1 Cross-sectional anatomy of the mid-portion of the left lower leg depicting the four compartments that must be released when performing a lower leg fasciotomy

The Lateral Incision of the Lower Leg

The lateral incision (Fig. 20.2) is made approximately 1.5–2 cm in front of the fibula and should, in general, extend from 5 cm below the head of the fibula down to 5 cm above the lateral malleolus. The exact length of the skin incision will depend on the clinical setting, but care must be taken to make sure that it is long enough that the constricting bands in the skin are divided. The skin and subcutaneous tissue are incised to expose the fascia encasing the lateral and anterior compartments. Care should be taken to avoid the lesser saphenous vein and peroneal nerve when making these skin incisions [5] (Fig. 20.3).

Once the skin flap is raised, the intermuscular septum is sought and identified. This is the structure that divides the anterior and lateral compartments. In the swollen or injured extremity, it may be difficult to find the intermuscular septum. In these circumstances, the septum can often be found by following the perforating vessels down to it (Fig. 20.4). Classically, the fascia of the lower leg is opened using an "H"-shaped incision (Fig. 20.5). This will be accomplished by making the cross piece of the "H" using a scalpel, which will expose both compartments and the septum. The legs of the "H" are made with curved Metzenbaum scissors using just the tips, which are turned away from the septum to avoid injury to the peroneal nerve (Fig. 20.5). It is important to identify the intermuscular septum and open the fascia at least 1 centimeter from it on either side, because the terminal branch of the deep peroneal nerve perforates the septum in the distal one-third of the lower leg, and this could be cut if care is not taken. The anterior and lateral compartments are then fasciotomized 1 cm in front and behind the intermuscular septum [5].

The fascia should be opened by pushing the partially opened scissor tips in both directions on either side of the septum, opening the fascia from the head of the fibula down to the lateral malleolus in a line that is 1–2 cm from the septum. Inspection of the septum and identification of the deep peroneal nerve and/or the anterior tibial vessels will confirm the entry into the anterior compartment. The skin incision should be closely inspected and extended as needed to ensure that its ends do not serve as a point of constriction.

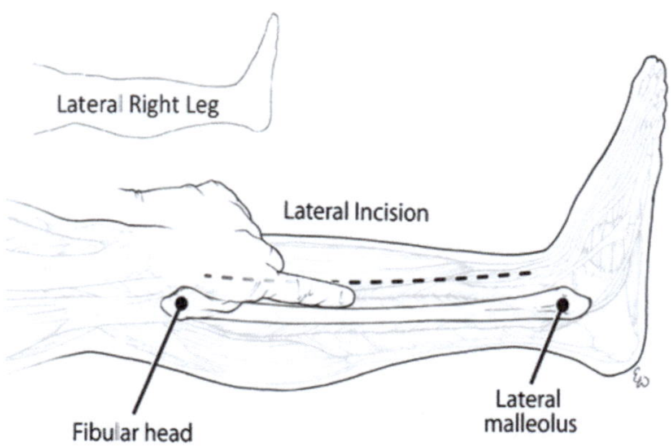

Fig. 20.2 The fibular head and lateral malleolus are reference points to mark the edge of the fibula, and the lateral incision (*dotted line*) is made one finger in front of this. One finger in front of the fibula

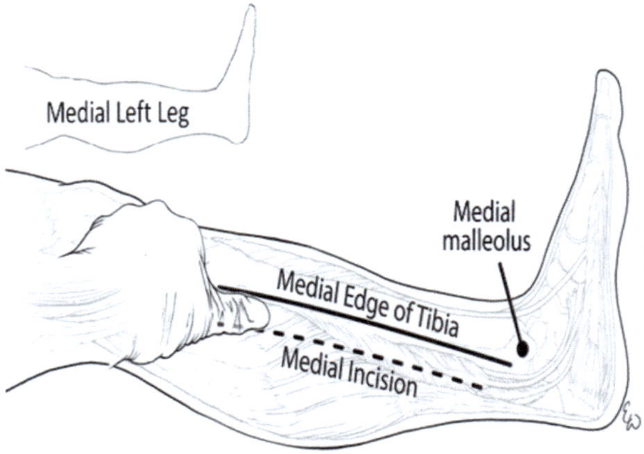

Fig. 20.3 The medial incision (*dotted line*) is made one thumb breadth below the palpable medial edge of the tibia (*solid line*). A thumb below the tibia

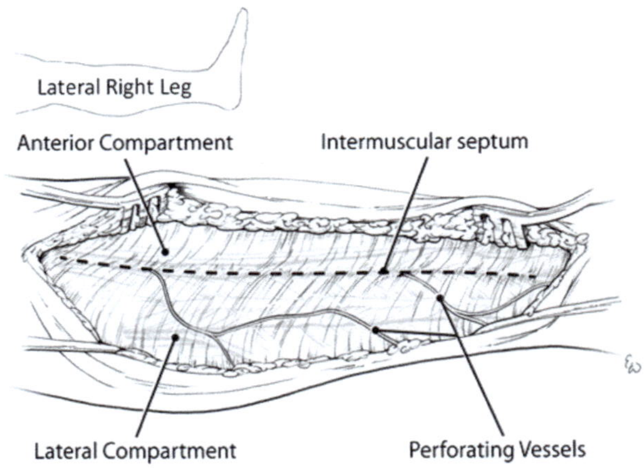

Fig. 20.4 The intermuscular septum separates the anterior and lateral compartments and is where the perforating vessels traverse. This is a representation of the lateral incision of the right lower leg

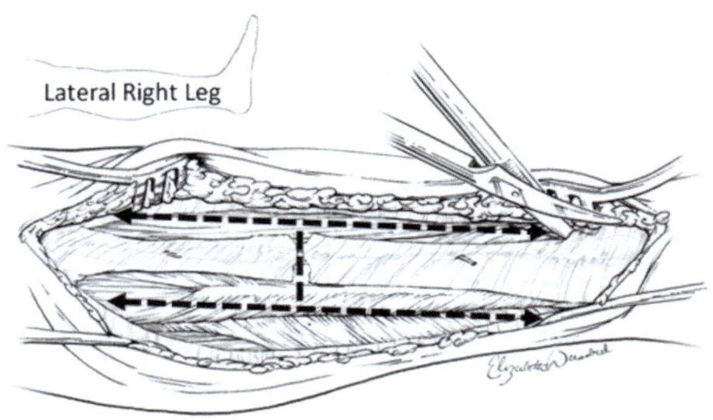

Fig. 20.5 The fascia overlying the anterior and lateral compartments is opened in a "H"-shaped fashion using scissors with the tips turned away from the intramuscular septum

The anterior compartment is the one most missed during lower extremity fasciotomy. One of the reasons for missing the anterior compartment stems from making the incision too far posteriorly, either directly over or behind the fibula. When the incision is made in this manner, the septum between the lateral and the superficial

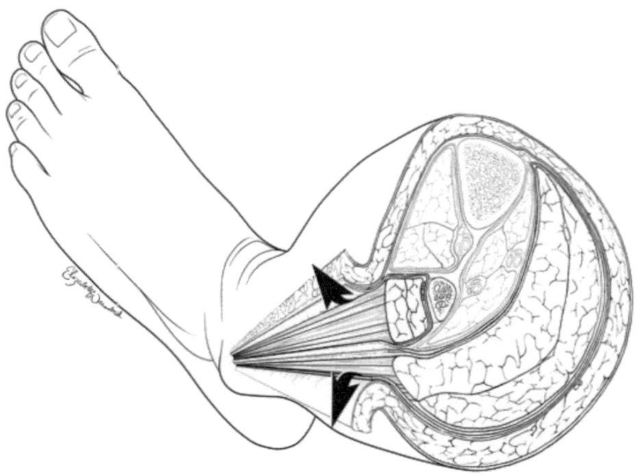

Fig. 20.6 When the lateral incision is made too far posterior, the septum between the lateral and superficial posterior compartments may be mistaken for that between the anterior and lateral leading to the anterior compartment not being opened

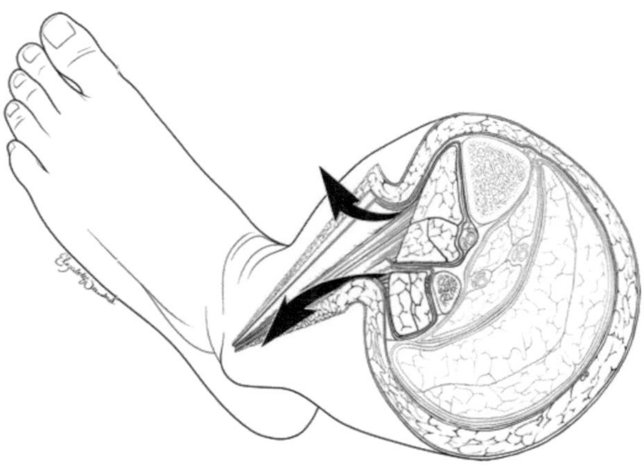

Fig. 20.7 When the lateral incision is made one finger in front of the fibula, the septum between the anterior and lateral compartments is more readily identified allowing for adequate decompression of both the anterior and lateral compartments

compartment may be directly below the incision and is sometimes erroneously identified as the septum between the anterior and lateral compartments (Fig. 20.6). When the lateral incision is made 1.5–2.0 cm in front of the fibula, the intramuscular septum between the anterior and lateral compartments is found directly below the incision making successful decompression likely (Fig. 20.7).

The Medial Incision of the Lower Leg

The medial incision is made 1.5–2.0 cm below the palpable medial edge of the tibia (Fig. 20.3). When making this incision, it is important to both identify and preserve the greater saphenous vein, as well as ligate any perforators to it, since these can bleed profusely. After dividing the skin and subcutaneous tissues, the fascia overlying the superficial posterior compartment, which contains the soleus and gastrocnemius muscle, is exposed. The fascia should be opened with a partially opened scissors from the tibial tuberosity to the medial malleolus to effectively decompress this compartment. The key to entering the deep posterior compartment is the soleus muscle. The soleus muscle attaches to the medial edge of the tibia, and dissecting these fibers (the soleal line and "soleus bridge") completely free from and exposing the underside of the tibia ensures entry into the deep posterior compartment (Fig. 20.8). Identification of the posterior tibial neurovascular bundle confirms that the compartment has been entered.

The deep posterior compartment can also be missed, and thorough understanding of the anatomy is the key to ensuring that this does not happen. One potential way to miss the deep posterior compartment is to get into the plane between the gastrocnemius and soleus muscle and believe that the compartment pressure has been released (Fig. 20.9). Proper decompression of the deep posterior compartment requires that the soleus fibers be separated from their attachment on the posterior surface of the tibia (Figs. 20.8 and 20.10).

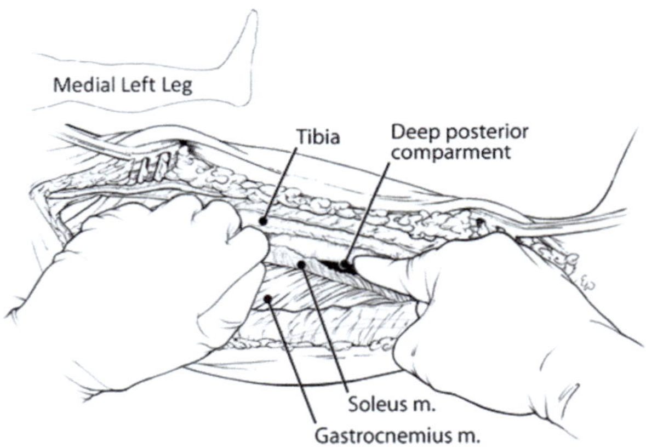

Fig. 20.8 The deep posterior compartment is entered by taking the soleus fibers down off the underside of the tibia

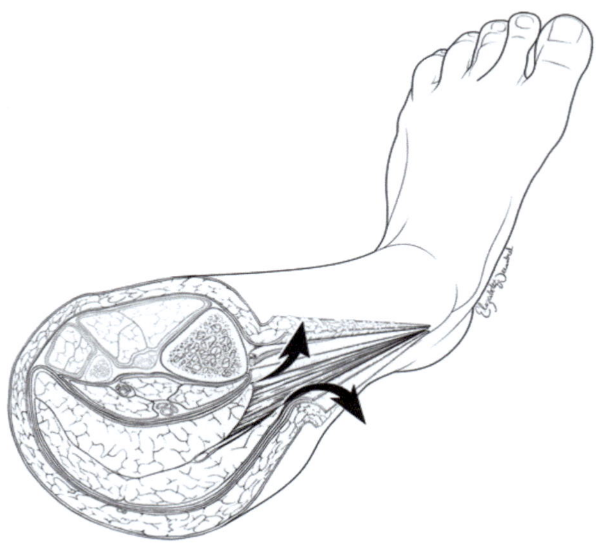

Fig. 20.9 A potential pitfall when doing the medial incision is to develop a plane between the gastrocnemius and soleus muscles and believing that this represents the plane between the superficial and deep posterior compartment

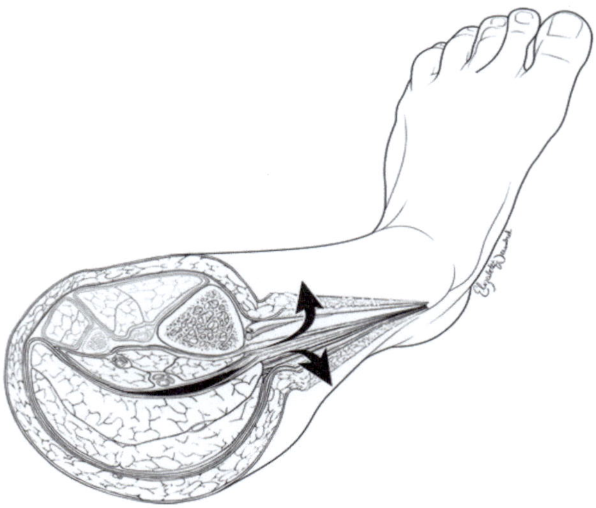

Fig. 20.10 Entry into and release of the deep posterior compartment require separating both the gastrocnemius and soleus from the underside of the tibia. Identification of the neurovascular bundle confirms that the deep posterior compartment has been entered

Wound Care

The muscle in each compartment should be assessed for viability. Viable muscle is pink and contracts when stimulated and bleeds when cut. Dead muscle should be debrided back to healthy viable tissue when necessary. Generally, fasciotomy wounds are not closed at the time of the initial procedure. These wounds are often large, and tissue swelling, skin retraction, or tissue loss make these wounds impossible to close at the initial setting, and closure would also defeat the release of pressure obtained by fasciotomy.

Wound management focuses on swelling control, allowing recovery of injured tissues and minimizing skin retraction. Patients are generally returned to the operating room every 24 to 72 h for dressing changes, reevaluation of muscle viability, and gradual closure of the wound. If the wounds cannot be primarily closed within 7–10 days, split-thickness skin grafts (STSG) may be required when both the patient and the wound are stable. Several techniques have been described to minimize skin retraction and obviate the need for STSG.

Both the vessel loop or shoelace technique and subatmospheric (negative pressure) wound dressings (e.g., wound VAC™, Kinetic Concepts, Inc (KCI), San Antonio, TX) have been used successfully to provide fasciotomy and open-wound control [5]. Both techniques are safe, reliable, and effective, though in small randomized studies, VAC™-treated wounds required longer time for closure with higher associated costs [5]. Other observational studies have failed to show superiority of modalities used in achieving earlier closure, or have shown the superiority of VAC over traditional wet-to-dry dressings, highlighting that there is unresolved controversy as to the ideal management of these wounds [5].

Complications

Patients with open fasciotomy wounds are at risk for infection, and incomplete or delayed fasciotomies can lead to permanent nerve damage, loss of limb, multisystem organ failure, rhabdomyolysis, and death. If muscle injury is extensive, either from prolonged ischemia or from direct crush, significant amounts of myoglobin may be released as the muscle is reperfused after fasciotomy. Early recognition and aggressive fasciotomy will help to minimize these adverse outcomes.

Rush and colleagues reported on a retrospective series of 127 lower extremity fasciotomies performed for CS after acute ischemia and revascularization in subjects with either vascular trauma or arterial occlusive disease [6]. Superficial infections occurred in five subjects, and all were resolved with local wound care. In their series, no limb loss was attributed to primary open fasciotomy [6]. They concluded that the morbidity and mortality of fasciotomy were the result of refractory ischemia caused by associated injuries or underlying medical problems, but not from open fasciotomy wound complications [6].

Invited Commentary

Ravi Rajani, MD, FACS

Despite decades of investigative work, the timely and consistent diagnosis of lower extremity compartment syndrome remains a challenge. It requires an attentive clinician with a constant high index of suspicion, which is particularly difficult in an era of ever-increasing demands on a physician's time with ever-decreasing ability to spend time directly at the bedside. As a result of these external factors, attempts have been made to "automate" the diagnosis, using objective measures, when possible, to replace or supplement clinical evaluation. Examples include tissue oximetry, scoring systems, and guidance by risk factors alone.

Absolute compartment pressure remains the most described objective measure, with a value of 30 mmHg historically chosen as a cutoff. This absolute number, however, may not be the correctly measured variable. Rather, the perfusion pressure, defined as the difference between the patient's diastolic blood pressure and the compartment pressure, may be a better choice, as it may more closely reflect changes in pressure which could lead to tissue damage. This "delta" pressure is well described and may serve as appropriate guidance in patients with unreliable clinical evaluations—for example, those who are intubated or with otherwise altered sensorium.

Lastly, any discussion of fasciotomies must also acknowledge the medicolegal issues at play. Missed compartment syndrome is a significant cause of litigation, and fear of such litigation may play a role in management decisions as providers adopt a defensive strategy "just in case." The complications of fasciotomy described herein must be kept in mind as surgeons balance the decision to proceed with compartment release—particularly in a prophylactic fashion. Increased length of stay, risk of nerve injury, and risk of infection have significant impacts on the patient's long-term outcome.

References

1. Abouezzi Z, Nassoura Z, Ivatury RR, et al. A critical reappraisal of indications for fasciotomy after extremity vascular trauma. Arch Surg. 1998;133(5):547–51.
2. Frykberg ER. Popliteal vascular injuries. Surg Clin North Am. 2002;82(1):67–89.
3. Kluckner M, Gratl A, Gruber L, et al. Predictors for the need for fasciotomy after arterial vascular trauma of the lower extremity. Injury. 2021;52(8):2160–5.
4. Wheeless CR, Fasciotomy of the leg. Wheeless' Textbook of Orthopaedics, 2020. https://www.wheelessonline.com/bones/fasciotomy-of-the-leg/. Accessed 4 Oct 2024.
5. Bowyer MW. Lower extremity fasciotomy: indications and technique. Curr Trauma Rep. 2015;1(1):35–44.
6. Rush DS, Frame SB, Bell RM, Berg EE, Kerstein MD, Haynes JL. Does open fasciotomy contribute to morbidity and mortality after acute lower extremity ischemia and revascularization? J Vasc Surg. 1989;10(3):343–50.

Lower Extremity Major Amputations 21

Transmetatarsal amputation (TMA) is a practical solution for the management of distal nonviable foot. The operation was popularized by McKittrick in 1949 and a few years later by Pederson and Day in 1954 [1]. The indication for TMA includes gangrene or infection involving multiple digits or involving the great toe. Amputation (TMA) can also be considered for gangrene extending a short distance on the dorsal skin, past the metatarsal phalangeal crease, provided that the plantar skin is viable. Contraindications include forefoot infection, cellulitis, and dependent rubor involving the dorsal aspect of the foot proximal to metatarsal phalangeal crease. Whenever possible, it is better to preserve the bases of all metatarsals. A more proximal level of amputation will result in a loss of the insertion of tibialis anterior with resulting equinus contracture (deformity) limiting the upward movement of the ankle joint and making it difficult to pull the foot up. This results in difficulty climbing stairs, walking, and getting in and out of cars. People with equinus deformity exhibit toe walking wherein the foot remains in a downward position during gait, while those with foot drop have a high stepping gait [1].

Below-knee Amputations (BKA)

Clinical examination of the condition of the skin below the knee is extremely useful in determining the healing of the below-the-knee stump. The healing potential of the skin at the amputation level is dependent on the vascularity at the level of amputation. Less than 25% of BKAs healed when a femoral pulse was absent. Furthermore, significantly more energy is required to ambulate with an above-knee prosthesis (50–70%) compared to those below-the-knee (10–40%) [2]. Considering these factors, on occasion, endovascular or even open arterial reconstruction might be necessary to ensure that the planned BKA will have adequate perfusion particularly in patients with contralateral AK amputation. Evolving from the earliest forms of amputations which were done predominantly for wounded warriors, trauma is less often an indication for amputation except in unsalvageable limbs. The most

S. S. Hans, *Contemporary Management of Lower Extremity Aneurysmal Disease*,
https://doi.org/10.1007/978-3-032-00159-7_21

common indications for below-knee amputation are critical limb ischemia and diabetes with infected gangrene. A large portion of amputations, that is, 82%, are done due to ischemia, despite aggressive thrombectomies or repeated arterial reconstructions [2]. In cases of severe infection, active cellulitis first needs to be controlled prior to amputation. If infection and necrosis are severe, a guillotine amputation is performed 2–3 cm above the ankle for source control, followed by a more definitive below-knee amputation, 5–7 days later. The level of amputation should be decided on after assessing the level of pathology, the potential for rehabilitation, and the presence of adequate perfusion [3, 4].

Pertinent Surgical Anatomy

There are four fascial compartments in the lower leg (Fig. 21.1): (1) Anterior compartment, laying anteromedial to the tibiofibular interosseous membrane, contains the tibialis anterior, extensor halluces longus, extensor digitorum longus, peroneus tertius, anterior tibial artery and vein, as well as deep peroneal nerve running alongside the vessels. The anterior tibial artery is the main blood supply to the anterior compartment, aided by the perforating branch of peroneal artery. (2) The lateral compartment, laying posterior to the anterior compartment and lateral to the fibula, contains peroneus longus, peroneus brevis, and the superficial peroneal nerve. (3) The posterior superficial compartment contains the soleus, gastrocnemius, and plantaris muscles. (4) The deep posterior compartment contains tibialis posterior, plantar flexors of the foot and toes, the tibial nerve, and the posterior tibial artery which supplies this compartment.

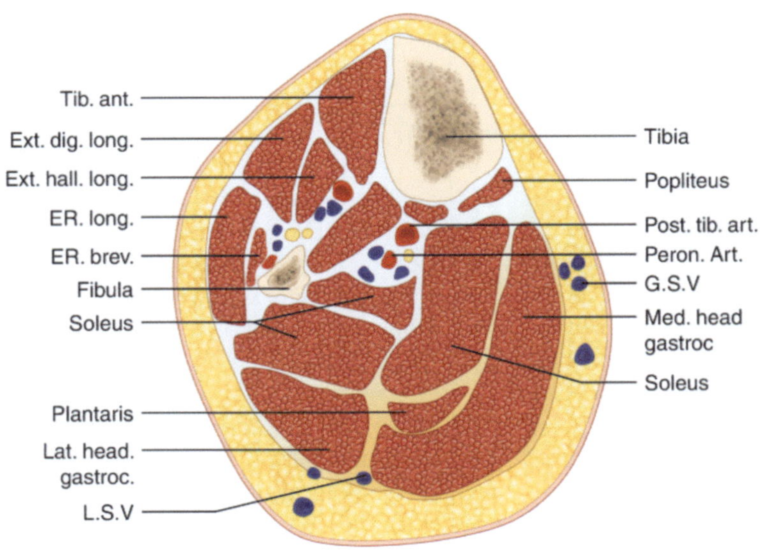

Fig. 21.1 Cross-sectional anatomy of the below-knee lower extremity

Guillotine amputation While several techniques can be adopted to perform the guillotine amputation, the goal is to ensure source control. The initial step is simply making a circumferential incision just proximal to the malleoli. Any patent-named vessels are suture ligated. The ligamentous attachments of the ankle are incised, exposing the periosteum of the tibia and fibula. The periosteum is elevated, and a saw is used to divide the bones. Electrocautery can be used to ensure hemostasis. Cultures can be sent to the microbiology lab, and dressings are applied. Definitive revision can take place in 5–7 days.

Preoperative Preparation

- Nutritional optimization to ensure healing.
- Cardiopulmonary risk stratification and optimization when feasible.
- General or regional anesthesia.
- Prophylactic antibiotics to reduce wound infection rates.
- Venous thromboembolism prophylaxis. There is an estimated 12.5% risk of venous thromboembolism in the perioperative period.
- Use of tourniquet is associated with a decrease in intraoperative blood loss. The patients requiring amputation for vascular disease commonly have associated occlusion of infrapopliteal arteries.

Operative Techniques

Skin incision (Fig. 21.2): The skin at the planned site of incision must be healthy without infection, breakdown, or ischemia. The most common technique is the long posterior flap. The anterior skin incision typically extends two-thirds of the circumference of the leg. This is made at least 10–12 cm or four fingerbreadths distal to the tibial tuberosity, which is the level at which the tibia is transected. Although a longer stump may aid functionally, functional stumps are achieved with as little as 5 cm of residual tibia. A thicker posterior flap aids in vascularity although it can have

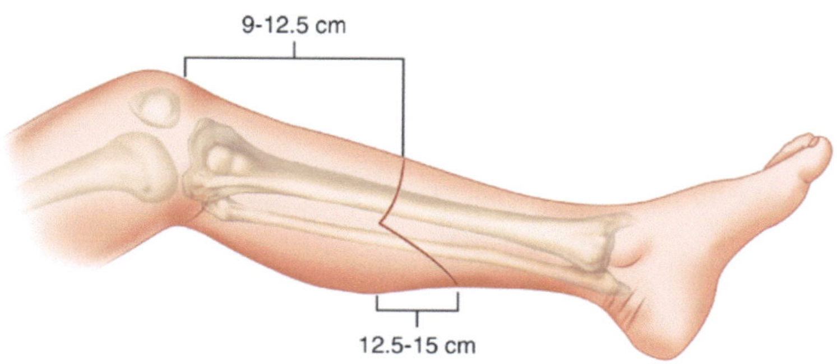

Fig. 21.2 BKA skin incision

cosmetic hitches while approximating the incision. Although various alternative flaps are described, the posterior flap is easy to construct and offers adequate coverage and padding of the stump. The length of the posterior flap should be 5–6 in or longer to ensure tension-free closure of the stump.

Neurovascular ligation (Fig. 21.3a): Understanding anatomy is of the utmost importance to anticipate and ligate structures appropriately. Major vessels are suture ligated, including anterior tibial, posterior tibial, and peroneal arteries. Large nerves are grasped, advanced, tied, transected, and allowed to retract into the depths of the wound to avoid neuroma formation.

Division of tibia and fibula (Fig. 21.3b): The periosteum of the tibia is elevated circumferentially proximally for 2 cm using a periosteal elevator and divided using a powered oscillating saw or a Gigli saw perpendicular to the axis of the tibia. The anterior edge of the tibia is then bevelled to eliminate sharp edges that can protrude through the skin. The fibula is transected using a saw or bone cutter 1–2 cm proximal to the tibia. Excessively short fibula can result in a conical stump that is difficult to fit with a prosthesis. However, excessively long fibula will be functionally inept.

Stump closure (Fig. 21.4a, b): Hemostasis should be ensured. Stump closure is in two layers, an interrupted layer of absorbable suture for fascia and interrupted loose nylon sutures for skin approximation to avoid skin ischemia. The stump is then placed in padded dressing.

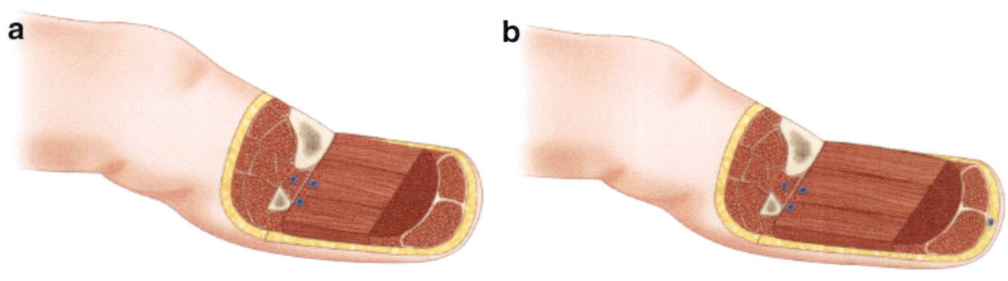

Fig. 21.3 (**a**) BKA: At the end of neurovascular ligation. (**b**) BKA: At the end of the division of tibia and fibula

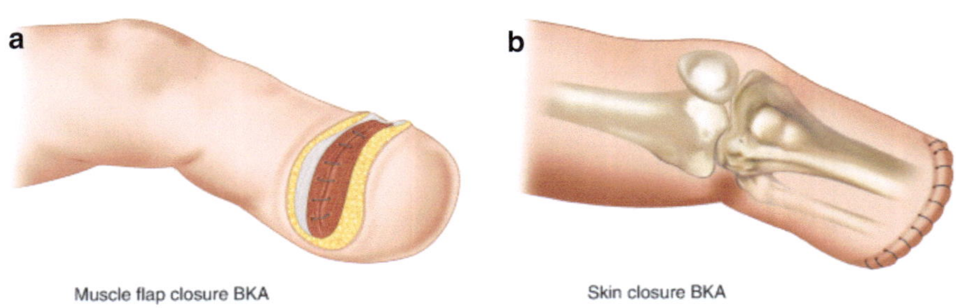

Fig. 21.4 (**a**, **b**) BKA: Stump closure

Potential Complications

- Inappropriate stump length.
- Flexion contracture of the knee following BKA—This can be prevented with knee immobilization in neutral position in immediate postoperative period and early rehabilitation.
- Hematoma, if significant especially in early postoperative period, should be evacuated in order to avoid a nidus for infection. If a tourniquet is used, the stump should be inspected after release of tourniquet for 5–10 min to avoid the potential of bleeding in the recovery room.
- Wound complications can include breakdown secondary to ischemia and wound infection. Wound infections are more common when amputations are performed on patients with infected gangrene and in patients with risk factors such as diabetes, malnutrition, malignancy, wound hematoma, and a prior history of arterial reconstruction with the use of prosthetic grafts.
- Stump ischemia can manifest as pallor, persistent pain, coolness of the stump, and progression to skin blisters and eventual necrosis. This results from lack of adequate vascularity or constrictive dressings. Stump trauma can occur secondary to pressure-induced necrosis from underlying bone or tourniquet-type dressing or shear injury.
- Furthermore, about 10–20% of patients eventually undergo above-knee amputations. Up to 30% of amputations can have wound complications. The estimated mortality at 3 years after an amputation is up to 43%.

Above-knee Amputation (AKA)

Indications

The most common indications for AKA include acute limb ischemia, chronic limb ischemia, and infection [5]. Some other AKA indications include trauma and malignancy. AKAs are performed in patients with irreversible acute limb ischemia, chronic limb ischemia after failed repeated revascularizations, patients with persistent severe chronic limb ischemia, and patients with BKA complications. Literature suggests that the mortality rate associated with major amputation exceeds that for revascularization, although this could be related to an implicit selection bias. Nehler et al. provide a qualitative approach indicating amputation over revascularization for patients with extensive severity in two of these three categories: comorbidities (notably diabetes and end-stage renal disease), complexity of revascularization, and the extent of tissue loss [6]. Approximately, 95% of AKAs heal compared to 80% of BKAs. An estimated 70% more energy is expended to walk on an AKA prosthesis compared to 40% on a BKA prosthesis. A palpable femoral pulse usually predicts AKA healing.

Pertinent Surgical Anatomy

The thigh is divided into anterior, posterior, and medial compartments (Fig. 21.5). The anterior compartment contains the vastus medius, vastus lateralis, vastus intermedius, rectus femoris, and genu articularis. Branches of the femoral nerve supply the anterior compartment. The sartorius runs anterior proximally to medial as it inserts distally onto the proximal tibia as a part of the pes anserinus. The saphenous nerve, a cutaneous branch of the femoral nerve, supplies the medial skin of the thigh and leg. The medial compartment contains the adductor magnus, adductor longus, adductor brevis, and gracilis. While the adductor magnus receives innervation from sciatic as well as obturator nerves, the rest of the medial compartment muscles are innervated by the obturator nerve. The medial compartment contains the femoral artery and vein which pass through the adductor hiatus to course posteriorly. The femoral artery provides blood flow to the muscles of the thigh and the femoral shaft through deep branches. The posterior compartment contains the long and short heads of biceps femoris, semitendinosus, semimembranosus, and the sciatic nerve which supplies this compartment. The great saphenous vein runs superficially along the medial aspect of the thigh.

Operative Techniques

- Skin incision (Fig. 21.6): A tourniquet can be used when there is sufficient salvageable femur length. The junction of the middle and distal thirds is the most common site of femur transection. Although many incisions are described, a transverse fishmouth incision with equal anterior and posterior flaps is

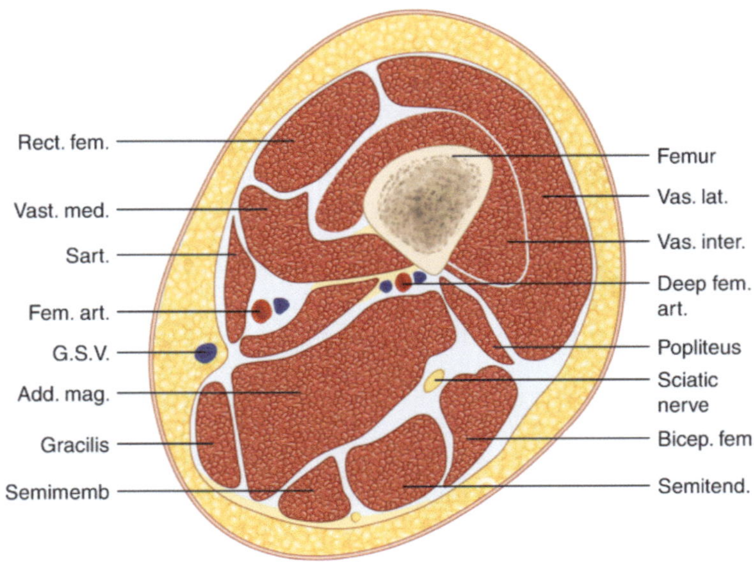

Fig. 21.5 AKA: Surgical anatomy

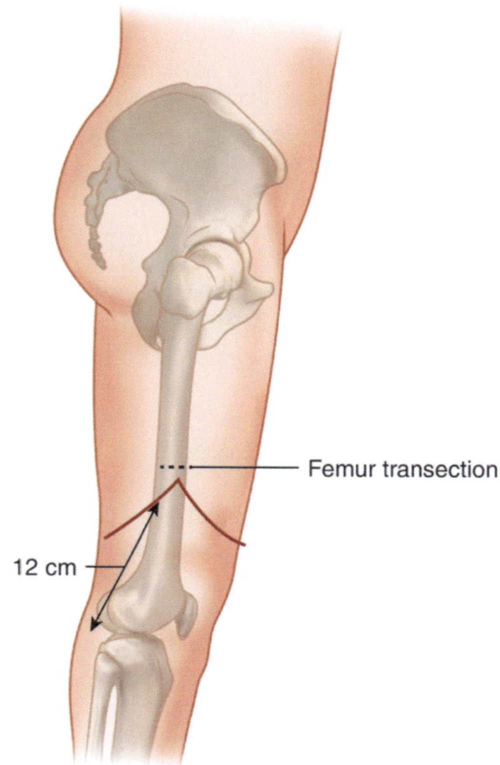

Fig. 21.6 AKA: Skin incision and transection of the femur

commonly used. Alternatives include circular incision with progressive layer deepening to the bone or sagittal flaps.

- Superficial femoral artery and vein are identified and suture ligated.
- Division of femur (Fig. 21.6): The femur is transected proximal to the skin incision using an oscillating saw; the edges are shaped to reduce pressure necrosis of the skin. Bone wax can be used to control bleeding from the marrow.
- Sciatic nerve is identified, sharply divided under tension, ligated, and allowed to retract into the deeper tissue.
- Wound closure: Stabilization of adductors by myopexy to avoid abduction and flexion of the proximal femur may be beneficial, though not commonly done for vascular pathology. Myopexy is performed by sewing the muscles of the posterior and medial compartment to the periosteum anterolateral to the femur. Deep fascia is approximated using absorbable suture. Skin is closed using interrupted monofilament sutures or staples which are removed in 4–6 weeks.

Postoperative Care

- Edema of the stump is an expected outcome, with an underappreciated component of the lymphatic edema. While some surgeons use vacuum-assisted dressings, some use rigid plaster dressings, and some use stump shrinkers to reduce this edema and wound complications that are associated with it. Elevation of the stump also reduces edema.
- Psychological support and targeted multimodal pain control are critical postoperatively. About 5% of patients experience phantom pain.
- Incision: Skin sutures are not removed until at least 2–3 weeks. A nonadherent gauze followed by dry dressing is typically used. Regular monitoring for wound complications is essential. Constrictive dressings must be avoided.

Potential Complications

- Hematoma, if significant, especially in early postoperative period, should be evacuated to avoid a nidus for infection.
- Wound complications, seen in up to 40% cases, can include breakdown secondary to ischemia and wound infection. Wound infections are more common when performed for infectious indications and in patients with risk factors such as diabetes, malnutrition, malignancy, wound hematoma, and prior prosthetic grafts. An aggressive approach to wound care must be adopted including liberal debridement, systemic antibiotics when appropriate, and nutritional optimization. Vacuum-assisted dressings can be particularly useful. In rare situations where local wound care is ineffective secondary to ischemia, aggressive attempts at revascularization should be performed as more proximal above-knee amputations can result in the same outcome as mid-transfemoral amputations.
- Stump ischemia can manifest as pallor, persistent pain, and coolness of the stump and may progress to skin blisters and eventual necrosis. This results from lack of adequate vascularity or constrictive dressings. Stump trauma can occur secondary to pressure-induced necrosis from underlying bone or tourniquet-type dressing or shear injury.
- Deep vein thrombosis and pulmonary embolism are seen in up to 50% patients after major lower extremity amputations. All patients should be on venous thromboembolic prophylaxis.
- Postoperative pain can be debilitating and could arise from the incision, ischemia, neuropathy, phantom pain, or infection. Multimodal therapy including regional anesthesia can prove beneficial. Physical and mental rehabilitations are key to recovery.
- Mortality perioperatively after an AKA range from 11% to 18%, most commonly secondary to sepsis, pneumonia, and cardiac complications. The survival rate at 1 year is approximately 50%, and less than 10% of elderly patients can walk on a prosthesis.

Hip Disarticulation

Indications

Hip disarticulation refers to the removal of the entire lower extremity through the hip joint. Hip disarticulation, when performed, is most often used for the treatment of high-grade diaphyseal tumors distal to the lesser trochanter, sometimes after massive trauma, for arterial insufficiency, severe infections, massive decubitus ulcers, or certain congenital limb deficiencies [7]. Although prostheses are available, few patients can utilize them, and energy requirements to use a prosthesis have been estimated to be 200% of normal ambulation. Mortality rates vary between 0% and 44%.

Operative Procedure

1. Incision (Fig. 21.7): Equal anterior and posterior flaps are utilized. With the patient in the lateral decubitus position, an anterior racquet-shaped incision is made beginning one fingerbreadth medial to the anterior superior iliac spine and curving it distally and medially almost parallel with the inguinal ligament to the pubic tubercle, pubic bone, and a point on the medial aspect of the thigh 5 cm distal to the origin of the adductor muscles (two fingerbreadths distal to the ischial tuberosity). The posterior incision continues around the posterior thigh

Fig. 21.7 Disarticulation hip—skin incision

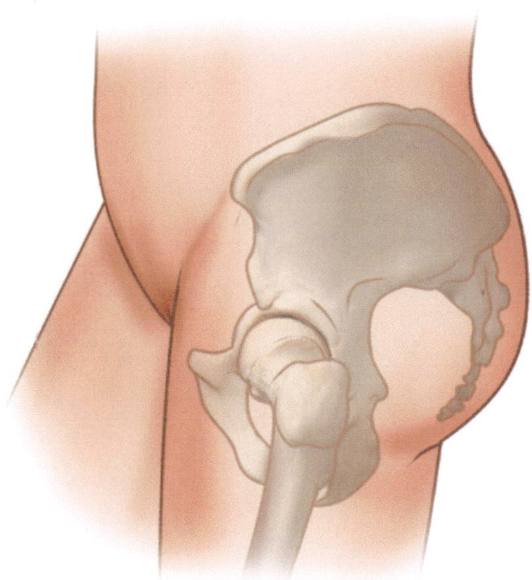

along the lateral aspect of the thigh about two fingerbreadths anterior to the greater trochanter.

If the buttock flap is extremely thick, the anterior incision can be moved laterally. The distance distal to the gluteal crease is directly proportional to the anterior-posterior diameter of the pelvis to allow for appropriate approximation of the flaps.

2. Femoral triangle exposure (Fig. 21.8): The skin, subcutaneous tissue, and Scarpa's fascia are dissected till the external oblique aponeurosis is identified. The superficial epigastric artery, branches of external pudendal artery, and branches of saphenous vein are divided and ligated. While the superficial inguinal lymph nodes are included in the specimen, the spermatic cord and round ligament are not.
3. Division of femoral vessels (Fig. 21.9): The femoral vessels are double ligated and transected. The femoral nerve is placed on gentle traction and ligated so that when divided, it retracts beneath the external oblique aponeurosis, so that if a neuroma forms, it will not be in a weight-bearing portion of the stump.
4. Division of muscles (Figs. 21.10 and 21.11): The sartorius is detached from the anterior superior iliac spine and rectus femoris from the anterior inferior iliac spine. The femoral sheath posterior to the femoral vessels is also incised using electrocautery to expose the hip joint capsule.

   The hip is flexed slightly to relax the iliopsoas; this allows for blunt finger dissection around the muscle in a mediolateral fashion. The entire muscle is

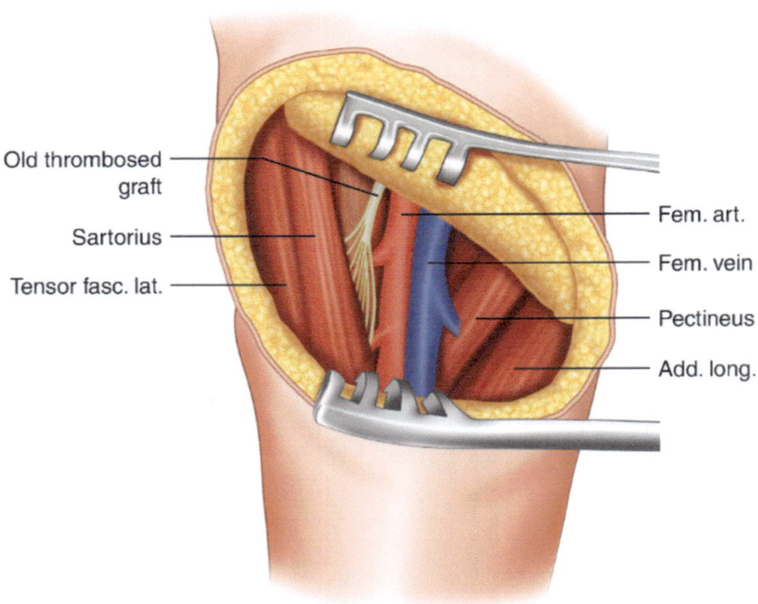

Fig. 21.8 Femoral triangle exposure

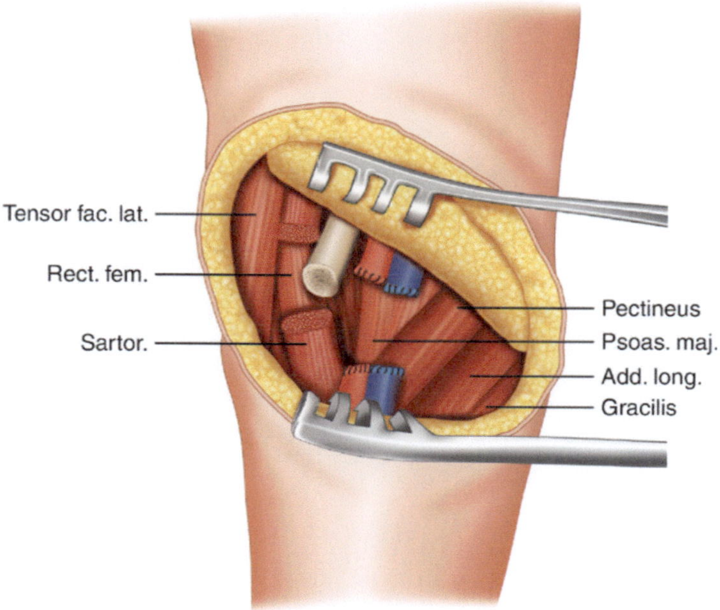

Fig. 21.9 Division of the femoral vessels

Fig. 21.10 Division of the muscles (sartorius, rectus femoris)

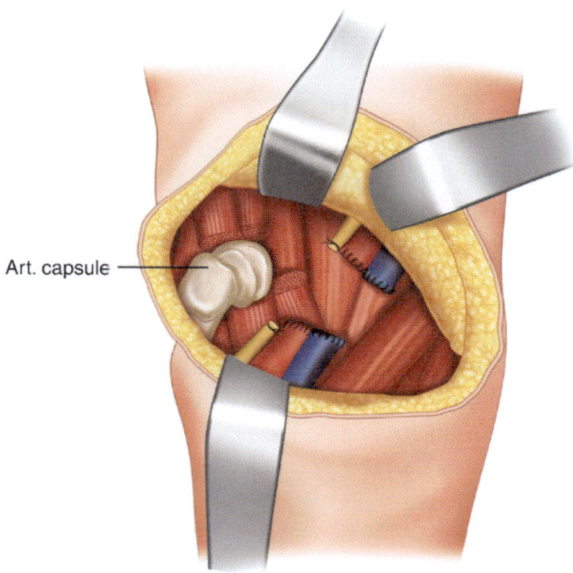

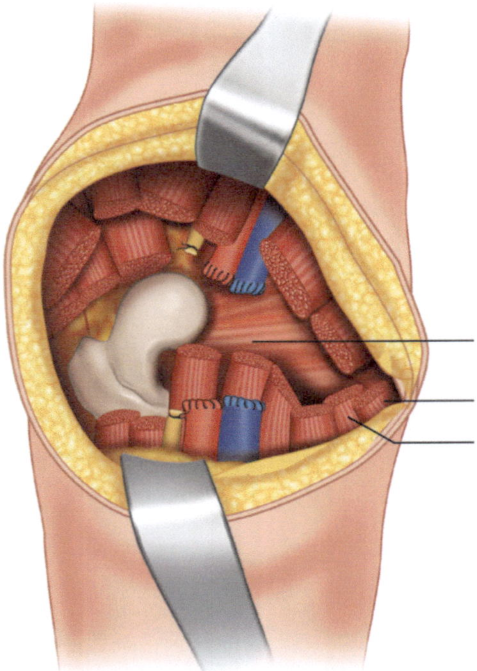

Fig. 21.11 Division of adductors and gracilis

dissected until the lesser trochanter is clearly identified while taking care to secure vessels that pass anterior to this muscle. The iliopsoas is divided at its insertion into the lesser trochanter.

- The adductors are then released from their origin on the pelvis. To preserve the obturator externus over the pelvis, its tendon arising from the lesser trochanter is identified to develop the plane between pectineus and obturator externus. A finger is passed beneath the pectineus, and it is released at its origin from the pubis using electrocautery. Beneath this, branches of the obturator artery, vein, and nerve are visualized.
- The adductor and gracilis muscles are detached from the pubis, and the part of the adductor magnus that arises from the ischium is divided at its origin. Obturator vessels and nerves are divided at this time. These bifurcate around the adductor brevis. The branches of the obturator artery should be carefully secured during dissection to prevent accidental rupture, retraction into the pelvis, and hemorrhage that is difficult to control. The abductor muscles are transected at their origin at the pubic symphysis.
- The obturator externus muscle is divided at its insertion on the femur instead of at its origin on the pelvis because otherwise the obturator artery may be severed and might retract into the pelvis, leading to hemorrhage that could be difficult to control.

5. Identification of the sciatic nerve (Fig. 21.12): The extremity is hyperabducted to help locate the ischial tuberosity. Cut ends of the abductor are retracted to find the tuberosity. Quadratus femoris, flexors, and sciatic nerve are identified. The quadratus femoris and the sciatic nerve are preserved. The semimembranosus, semitendinosus, and the long head of the biceps are transected at their origin from the ischial tuberosity. *Care should be taken to avoid the circumflex femoral vessels.*

   At this point, all anterior and posterior muscle groups have been divided. The joint capsule overlying the head of the femur is incised, and the ligamentum teres transected.
6. Posterior skin incision, transection of tensor fascia lata, gluteus maximus: The patient's torso is tilted posterolateral to anterolateral position. The skin incision posteriorly is taken down through the gluteal fascia. The tensor fascia lata and gluteus maximus are divided (neither at the origin nor at the insertion).

   Once the gluteus maximus is divided (Fig. 21.13), the common tendon containing multiple muscles—gluteus medius, gluteus minimus, piriformis, superior gemellus, obturator internus, inferior gemellus, and quadratus femoris—that insert into the greater trochanter is exposed, and these muscles are divided close to their insertion into the point.
7. Release of the specimen: The posterior portion of the joint capsule is incised. The sciatic nerve is dissected free, transected high near the sciatic notch, and allowed to retract beneath the piriformis.
8. Closure (Fig. 21.14) must consist of tenodesing the remaining muscles over the acetabulum.

   The obturator externus and gluteus medius are approximated over the joint capsule of the acetabulum to provide soft tissue coverage of bony prominences. The gluteal fascia is then elevated and approximated to the inguinal ligament and the pubic ramus. Sutures are placed bisecting the fascial edge uniformly prior to being tied as the posterior myocutaneous flap is much longer than the anterior fascia. Subfascial drains are placed prior to closure. The skin is closed over this. Subcutaneous drains can also be used prior to skin closure.

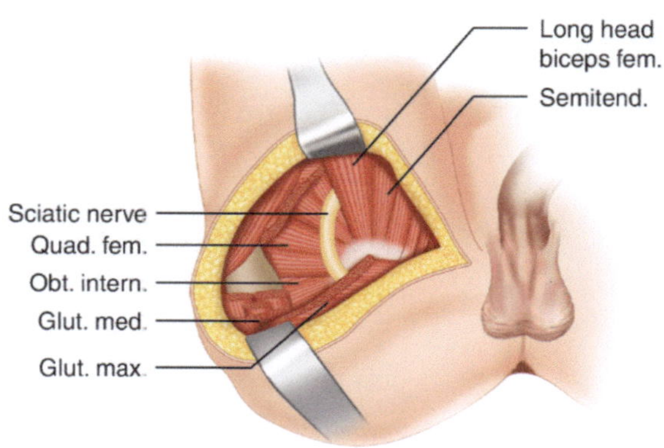

Fig. 21.12 Identification of the sciatic nerve

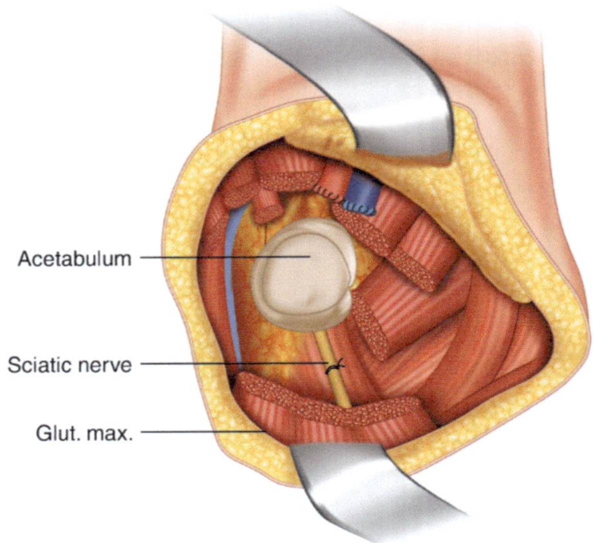

Fig. 21.13 Division of the gluteus maximus

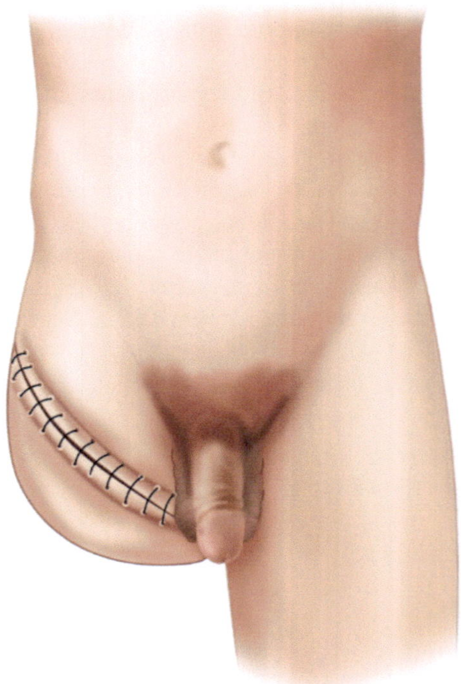

Fig. 21.14 Closure

Complications

Hip disarticulations are extremely invasive and mutilating procedures. Optimizing nutritional status and packed red cell transfusions when necessary are vital to reduce morbidity. In addition to thromboembolism, and debilitating pain seen in other major lower limb amputations, the morbidity and mortality seen with hip disarticulations are higher.

- Phantom limb: It is reported that patients who undergo hip disarticulations are 1.53 times more likely to experience phantom limb pain than patients who undergo below-knee amputations [8].
- Wound complications: Complication rates for hip disarticulation, including events such as infection, wound healing, and hematoma formation, have been reported to be as high as 60% [8]. Wound complications were more frequently noted in disarticulations performed for ischemic or infectious indications. Flap necrosis and wound sloughs are also common complications. Patients with a posterior flap, who had ligation of the common iliac vessels, were 2.7 times more likely to have flap necrosis than those patients who had ligation of the external iliac vessels. The extent of gluteal or flap dissection is quoted to have some bearing on flap necrosis.
- A 5-year mortality rate of 37–55% is reported when disarticulations are performed secondary to ischemia. Emergency situations have increased mortality as well, when compared to elective disarticulations. Generally, patients with hip disarticulations performed secondary to tumors have better outcomes.

Invited Commentary

Animesh Rathore, MD

This chapter provides a detailed overview of surgical procedures for major lower extremity amputations, including transmetatarsal, below-knee (BKA), above-knee (AKA), and hip disarticulations. It offers valuable insights into indications, techniques, and postoperative care, tailored to patients with severe vascular diseases, diabetes, or trauma-related complications.

The chapter begins with the historical context and indications for these surgeries, emphasizing the importance of vascular assessment to determine the level of amputation. Transmetatarsal amputations are highlighted as a function-preserving option for patients with localized foot gangrene, provided that adequate plantar skin remains viable. In contrast, the complexity of BKAs and AKAs underscores the balance between stump functionality, vascular health, and energy expenditure for prosthetic mobility.

Key surgical details are meticulously outlined, such as flap creation, neurovascular ligation, and the shaping of residual bones to enhance prosthetic compatibility. The emphasis on the understanding of the underlying surgical anatomy reflects the intricate nature of these procedures. Additionally, optimization of the preoperative factors of nutrition, infection prevention, and revascularization help with successful recovery from the operation. The narrative particularly shines in its discussion of BKA versus AKA, noting the increased energy demands and reduced mobility associated with above-knee prostheses.

Postoperative care and potential complications receive significant attention, with recommendations for wound care, infection prevention, and rehabilitation. Successful management following a major amputation involves collaborative care during the postoperative phase with the vascular specialists, prosthetists, physical therapist, as well as social worker. The inclusion of challenges like phantom limb pain and stump ischemia provides a comprehensive view of patient outcomes. The chapter's commentary on hip disarticulation adds depth by exploring its rare but critical use cases, often for malignancy or severe infections.

Overall, this chapter serves as a comprehensive guide, blending clinical precision with a patient-centered approach. Its thorough coverage of surgical techniques, combined with pragmatic discussions on rehabilitation and complications, makes it a valuable resource for vascular surgeons and multidisciplinary teams managing limb salvage and amputation cases.

References

1. Potti C, Peshkepija A. Lower extremity major amputations. In: Hans SS, Weaver MR, Nypaver TJ, editors. Primary and repeat arterial reconstructions. Cham: Springer International Publishing; 2023. p. 365–80.
2. McIntyre K. Below-knee amputation. In: Stanley JC, Veith F, Wakefield TW, editors. Current therapy in vascular and endovascular surgery. Philadelphia: Elsevier Health Sciences; 2014. p. 647–9.
3. O'Dwyer KJ, Edwards MH. The association between lowest palpable pulse and wound healing in below knee amputations. Ann R Coll Surg Engl. 1985;67(4):232–4. PMID: 4037633.
4. Eidt JF, Kalapatapu VR. Above and below-knee amputation. In: Atlas of vascular surgery and endovascular therapy. Philadelphia: Elsevier; 2014. p. 604–9.
5. Feezor R, Huber T. Above-knee amputation and hip disarticulation. In: Current therapy in vascular and endovascular surgery. 5th ed. Philadelphia: Saunders; 2014. p. 649–51.
6. Nehler MR, Coll JR, Hiatt WR, Regensteiner JG, Schnickel GT, Klenke WA, et al. Functional outcome in a contemporary series of major lower extremity amputations. J Vasc Surg. 2003;38(1):7–14. PMID: 12844082.
7. Sugarbaker PH, Chretien PB. A surgical technique for hip disarticulation. Surgery. 1981;90(3):546–53. PMID: 7268632.
8. Huffman A, Schneeberger S, Goodyear E, West JM, O'Brien AL, Scharschmidt TJ, et al. Evaluating hip disarticulation outcomes in a 51-patient series. J Orthop. 2022;31:117–20. PMID: 35541569.

22 Multiple-Choice Questions

Chapter 1: History of Lower Extremity Aneurysmal Disease

1. For the management of aneurysmal disease, which technique was advocated by Ambroise Paré?
   A. Direct compression therapy
   B. Ligation of aorta
   C. Proximal ligature
   D. Indirect compression therapy

Correct Answer: C

2. The first physician to treat leaking iliac artery aneurysm in a terminally ill patient was
   A. John Hunter
   B. Ambroise Paré
   C. Theodore Mannoir
   D. Astley Cooper

Correct Answer: D

3. The first successful treatment of popliteal aneurysm was performed by
   A. Theordore Matas
   B. John Hunter
   C. Andrew Gibson
   D. Alexis Carrel

Correct Answer: B

S. S. Hans, *Contemporary Management of Lower Extremity Aneurysmal Disease*,
https://doi.org/10.1007/978-3-032-00159-7_22

Chapter 2: Surgical Anatomy of the Lower Extremity Vascular System

1. The mean diameter of the common femoral artery is
   A. 10.5 mm in men and 9.5 mm in women
   B. 10.2 mm in men and 9.2 mm in women
   C. 9.8 mm in men and 8.2 mm in women
   D. 9.2 mm in men and 7.8 mm in women

Correct Answer: C

2. Persistent sciatic arteries are associated with aneurysm formation in more than
   A. 10% of cases
   B. 15% of cases
   C. 20% of cases
   D. 25% of cases

Correct Answer: D

3. High origin of anterior tibial artery is present in
   A. Less than 1% of cadaveric and angiographic studies
   B. 1.5–3% of cadaveric and angiographic studies
   C. 1.9–4.2% of cadaveric and angiographic studies
   D. 4.5–5.5% of cadaveric and angiographic studies

Correct Answer: C

4. The distal portion of the peroneal artery is overlapped by which muscle?
   A. Flexor digitorum longus
   B. Tibialis posterior
   C. Flexor hallucis longus
   D. Peroneus longus

Correct Answer: C

5. The great saphenous vein has
   A. 0–5 venous valves
   B. 5–9 venous valves
   C. 10–20 venous valves
   D. 21–25 venous valves

Correct Answer: C

Chapter 3: Duplex Sonography of Lower Extremity Aneurysmal Disease

1. Examination of superficially located arteries of the lower extremities is performed with a transducer frequency of
   A. 3 MHz
   B. 5 MHz
   C. 5–7.5 MHz
   D. 12 MHz

Correct Answer: C

2. True femoral artery aneurysms are more common in men with the ratio of men to women being
   A. 5:1
   B. 10:1
   C. 15:1
   D. 20:1

Correct Answer: B

3. Popliteal aneurysms are diagnosed with color duplex ultrasound with a transducer frequency of
   A. 3 MHz
   B. 4 MHz
   C. 5–7 MHz
   D. 8–10 MHz

Correct Answer: C

4. True femoral artery aneurysms are associated with aortic and iliac aneurysms in
   A. 60–62% cases
   B. 50–59% cases
   C. 41–49% cases
   D. 30% cases

Correct Answer: A

Chapter 4: MRA and CT Angiography of Lower Extremity Aneurysmal Disease

1. CTA should not be performed in patients with a GFR of
   A. 50–60 mL/min
   B. 45–49 mL/min
   C. 40–44 mL/min
   D. Less than 30 mL/min

Correct Answer: D

2. A patient with GFR of 38 mL/min is scheduled for CTA. The optimal strategy to reduce the incidence of contrast-induced nephropathy is
   A. Use of dopamine
   B. N-acetyl cysteine
   C. Hydration with the use of nonionic iso-osmolar agents (iodixanol) with the use of diluted contrast with a smaller volume
   D. Preprocedure hemodialysis

Correct Answer: C

3. Which study is preferable for definitive management of a large popliteal aneurysm in a patient with GFR of 30 mL/min?
   A. Color duplex imaging
   B. CTA
   C. MRA
   D. Catheter-based arteriography with the use of CO_2

Correct Answer: C

4. Contrast-enhanced MRA is more accurate than TOF MRA in the settings of
   A. Slow flow
   B. High-grade stenosis
   C. Fast flow in the presence of moderate stenosis
   D. Slow flow and high-grade stenosis

Correct Answer: D

5. Gadofosveset trisodium (contrast agent used for MRA) has an extended half-life in the distribution phase, which is up to
   A. 30 min
   B. 45 min
   C. 60 min
   D. 90 min

Correct Answer: C

Chapter 5: Catheter-Based Arteriography for Evaluation of the Lower Extremity Aneurysmal Disease

1. A patient with previous endograft (Excluder) for AAA repair needs catheter-based arteriography for selective evaluation of right popliteal artery aneurysm with associated infrapopliteal associated disease. The best access site is
   A. Right brachial
   B. Left brachial
   C. Retrograde right femoral
   D. Retrograde left femoral

Correct Answer: B

2. A severe anaphylactic reaction to iodine in patients receiving a nonionic contrast agent occurs in
   A. 1% of patients
   B. 0.5% of patients
   C. 0.2–0.4% of patients
   D. 0.04% of patients

Correct Answer: D

3. The incidence of access-related complications is reduced by
   A. Puncture using bony landmarks
   B. Puncture using bony landmark and use of micropuncture technique
   C. Using calcium in the arterial wall as a guide for puncture
   D. Use of a routine ultrasound for puncture

Correct Answer: D

4. Vascular closure devices as compared to manual compression have a
   A. Reduced access-related complications
   B. Less incidence of infections
   C. Increased safety
   D. Complication rates are comparable between vascular closure devices and manual compression.

Correct Answer: D

5. Radiation dose with DSA as compared to standard arteriography is
   A. Higher
   B. Same
   C. Lower
   D. Only higher if magnification is used

Correct Answer: A

Chapter 6: Degenerative Femoral Artery Aneurysms

1. The incidence of rupture of degenerative femoral artery aneurysm is
   A. 1%
   B. 2%
   C. 3–5%
   D. 6–8%

Correct Answer: B

2. The current guideline for repair of asymptomatic degenerative femoral artery aneurysm is when aneurysm reaches the Tr/AP diameter of
   A. 2.5 cm
   B. 2.6–3.0 cm
   C. 3.1–3.4 cm
   D. 3.5 cm or greater

Correct Answer: D

3. Common femoral artery aneurysm involving its bifurcation is best repaired by
   A. Endovascular technique with covered stent
   B. Interposition vein graft following resection
   C. Interposition synthetic graft following resection
   D. Interposition synthetic graft with reimplantation of profunda femoris artery or an interposition graft to profunda femoris artery

Correct Answer: D

4. Postoperative swelling after open repair of CFA aneurysm is caused by
   A. Reperfusion
   B. Venous obstruction
   C. Lymphatic disruption
   D. Hematoma in the groin

Correct Answer: C

5. A distal deep femoral artery aneurysm (profunda femoris) in a patient with patent SFA is best treated by
   A. Proximal ligation
   B. Stent graft
   C. Coil embolization
   D. Interposition graft

Correct Answer: C

Chapter 7: Femoral Artery Pseudoaneurysm Secondary to Femoral Artery Intervention and Penetrating Trauma

1. The incidence of femoral pseudoaneurysm following femoral access for coronary and peripheral diagnostic arteriography is
   A. 3–5%
   B. 2.1–2.9%
   C. 0.5–2.0%
   D. Less than 0.5%

Common Answer: C

2. A femoral pseudoaneurysm with a size of less than 2.0 cm is diagnosed by color DUS following diagnostic arteriography. Patient is not on any anticoagulation or antiplatelet medications. He has minimal groin discomfort. The optimal management consists of
   A. Observation and follow-up DUS in 1 week
   B. Ultrasonic compression
   C. Thrombin injection in the sac
   D. Operative repair

Correct Answer: A

3. Following peripheral arterial intervention, a 67-year-old man with morbid obesity complains of pain and swelling in the right groin with stable vital signs. He has no back pain. There is an audible bruit in the groin. Initial DUS does not show the presence of femoral pseudoaneurysm. The next best strategy is
   A. Obtain CTA
   B. Obtain MRA
   C. Increase the depth on ultrasound machine to greater than 4 cm
   D. Discharge the patient, and reassure him that there is no evidence of pseudoaneurysm

Correct Answer: C

4. Ultrasound-guided compression is associated with
   A. Increased time to achieve thrombosis
   B. Increased pain with ultrasound-guided compression
   C. Increased time and increased pain during the procedure
   D. More success than ultrasound-guided thrombin injection

Correct Answer: C

5. Success rate of ultrasound-guided thrombin injection for the treatment of a femoral pseudoaneurysm is
   A. 70–80%
   B. 81–85%
   C. 86–90%
   D. 91–100%

Correct Answer: D

Chapter 8: Femoral Artery Anastomotic Aneurysms

1. The incidence of femoral artery anastomotic aneurysm 15 years following aortofemoral reconstruction is approximately
   A. 25%
   B. 20%
   C. 15%
   D. 10%

Correct Answer: A

2. Coagulase-negative staphylococcal infection has been reported in what percentage of cases of femoral anastomotic aneurysms
   A. 30%
   B. 40%
   C. 50%
   D. 60%

Correct Answer: D

3. Femoral anastomotic aneurysms should be repaired in patients with a diameter greater than
   A. 3.5 cm
   B. 3.0 cm
   C. 2.5 cm
   D. 2.0 cm

Correct Answer: C

4. The most common complication of repair of femoral anastomotic aneurysm is
   A. Infection
   B. Hemorrhage
   C. Lymphatic leak, lymphocele
   D. Thrombosis

Correct Answer: C

5. Lymphocele following repair of femoral anastomotic aneurysm is best diagnosed by
   A. CT scan pelvis
   B. Lymphoscintigraphy
   C. MRI pelvis
   D. Color-duplex ultrasound

Correct Answer: A

Chapter 9: Complex Femoral Anastomotic Aneurysms

1. Most patients with leaking femoral anastomotic aneurysms present with
   A. Hypotension
   B. Severe back pain
   C. Groin pain, mass with ecchymosis in the groin and thigh
   D. Acute ischemia in the lower extremity

Correct Answer: C

2. In a patient with a leaking femoral anastomotic aneurysm 6 cm in diameter, proximal control should be obtained by
   A. A hockey-stick incision in the groin
   B. Transverse suprainguinal incision with exposure of the limb of the aorto-femoral graft
   C. Balloon occlusion using contralateral femoral access
   D. Balloon occlusion using left brachial access

Correct Answer: B

3. Recurrent femoral anastomotic aneurysms are more common in
   A. Men
   B. Women
   C. 4–5 years of aortofemoral grafting
   D. B, C, and a history of local wound complications such as infection

Correct Answer: D

4. The worst outcomes following repair of femoral anastomotic aneurysms are in those
   A. With large size FAAs with a diameter of 7.5 cm
   B. With recurrent femoral AAs
   C. Presenting with thrombosis
   D. Presenting with thrombosis and rupture

Correct Answer: D

Chapter 10: Mycotic Femoral Artery Aneurysms

1. The common causes of mycotic femoral artery aneurysms are
   A. Bacterial endocarditis
   B. Following femoropopliteal bypass using PTFE graft
   C. Following femoral artery access for severely infected ischemic ulcer in the foot
   D. Redo aortofemoral graft reconstruction

Correct Answer: A

2. Most mycotic femoral artery aneurysms are pseudoaneurysms and have the potential to cause
   A. Limb loss
   B. Secondary hemorrhage
   C. Sepsis
   D. Limb loss, secondary hemorrhage, and mortality

Correct Answer: D

3. Ligation of mycotic femoral artery at its bifurcation results in a limb loss with an incidence of greater than
   A. 50%
   B. 40%
   C. 30%
   D. 20%

Correct Answer: C

4. The best option for reconstruction following ligation/resection of a mycotic femoral aneurysm is
   A. Use of internal iliac artery as a graft
   B. Use of superficial femoral and popliteal vein
   C. Extra-anatomic obturator bypass
   D. Use of PTFE or rifampicin-soaked Daron graft as a lateral bypass over the iliac crest

Correct Answer: C

5. Mycotic femoral artery aneurysm in a patient with intravenous drug abuse is best managed by
   A. Ligation of femoral artery and immediate revascularization
   B. Ligation and definitive delayed revascularization
   C. Ligation, debridement, intravenous antibiotics, and delayed revascularization necessary only in small percentage of cases
   D. Ligation, debridement, intravenous antibiotics, evaluation of DP and PT Doppler flow in the foot, and if a flow signal is detected, revascularization should be avoided

Correct Answer: D

Chapter 11: Endovascular Repair of Popliteal Artery Aneurysms

1. The prevalence of popliteal artery aneurysms
   A. 4.4/100,000
   B. 5.4/100,000
   C. 6.39/100,000
   D. 7.39/100,000

Correct Answer: D

2. Due to development of thromboembolic complications, the risk of limb loss in a patient with popliteal aneurysm is
   A. 50%
   B. 40%
   C. 30%
   D. 20%

Correct Answer: B

3. Popliteal aneurysm should be repaired in a patient
   A. Diameter of 2 cm without thrombus
   B. Diameter of 2 cm with moderate amount of thrombus
   C. Diameter of 1.8 cm without thrombus
   D. Diameter of 1.5 cm without thrombus

Correct Answer: B

4. For endovascular repair of popliteal artery aneurysm, the normal length of proximal and distal landing zones should be
   A. 1.5 cm
   B. 2.0 cm
   C. 2.5 cm
   D. 3.0 cm

Correct Answer: B

5. For endovascular repair of popliteal aneurysm, the associate vessel tortuosity of ________ is acceptable
   A. Less than 30°
   B. Less than 25°
   C. Less than 40°
   D. Less than 45°

Correct Answer: D

6. In patients requiring multiple endografts for the endovascular repair of the popliteal aneurysms, the smaller device is placed first distally, and an overlap is maintained for a distance of
   A. 1–2 cm
   B. 2–3 cm
   C. 2.5–3.5 cm
   D. 3.6–4.0 cm

Correct Answer: B

Chapter 12: Open Repair of Popliteal Artery Aneurysms

1. Posterior approach for open repair of popliteal aneurysm is preferred in patients with location of the aneurysm
   A. Above the knee joint line
   B. At the knee joint line
   C. Below the knee joint line
   D. Starting at the level of adductor tubercle and extending to 3 inches below the knee joint

Correct Answer: B

2. The primary objective for repair of popliteal aneurysm is to
   A. Relieve pain
   B. Prevent rupture
   C. Prevent acute thrombosis
   D. Prevent acute thrombosis and distal embolization

Correct Answer: D

3. In order to expose bifurcation of the popliteal artery which muscle needs to be divided
   A. Sartorius
   B. Tendons of pes anserinus
   C. Soleus from soleal line
   D. Popliteus

Correct Answer: C

4. The risk of amputation following open repair with bypass of a popliteal aneurysm in an asymptomatic patient at 30 days is
   A. 0.5%
   B. 1.0%
   C. 1.4%
   D. 2.0%

Correct Answer: C

5. One-year patency of bypass with exclusion of popliteal aneurysm is
   A. 80% for GSV and 50% for synthetic graft
   B. 85% for GSVC and 55% synthetic graft
   C. 90% for GSV and 60% for synthetic graft
   D. 96% for GSV and 67% for synthetic graft

Correct Answer: D

Chapter 13: Management of Mycotic Popliteal Artery Aneurysms and Popliteal Pseudoaneurysm

1. The following statement best reflects the pathogenesis of mycotic aneurysm
   A. The normal arterial intima is susceptible to infection.
   B. The normal arterial intima is resistant to infection.
   C. The normal arterial intima is resistant to infection and is rarely affected unless the virulence of the organism is very high.
   D. The normal intima is resistant to infection and is rarely affected unless the virulence of the organism is very high or the patient is immunocompromised.

Correct Answer: D

2. Blood culture is positive in what percentage of patients with a mycotic popliteal aneurysm
   A. 30%
   B. 40%
   C. 50%
   D. 60%

Correct Answer: C

3. Following complete excision of a mycotic popliteal aneurysm and revascularization, the duration of antibiotics therapy should be
   A. Eight weeks of antibiotics with first 2 weeks by intravenous route
   B. Six weeks of antibiotics with first 3 weeks by intravenous route
   C. Six weeks of antibiotics with first 2 weeks by intravenous route
   D. Four weeks of antibiotics with first 2 weeks by intravenous route

Correct Answer: C

4. Following knee arthroplasty, a 76-year-old woman presents with symptomatic popliteal artery pseudoaneurysm, the best method of repair is
   A. Open repair
   B. Endovascular repair using coil embolization
   C. Ultrasound-guided thrombin injection
   D. Stent graft repair

Correct Answer: D

5. Mycotic popliteal aneurysm is best diagnosed by
   A. Clinical exam and elevated WBC count and positive blood culture
   B. Nuclear scan
   C. CT angiography
   D. Catheter-based angiography

Correct Answer: C

Chapter 14: Acute Thrombosis of the Popliteal Aneurysm

1. Acute thrombosis manifest in what percent of patients with popliteal aneurysms
   A. 15%
   B. 20%
   C. 23%
   D. 28%

Correct Answer: D

2. A 67-year-old man presents to the ER with Rutherford II A ischemia due to acute thrombosis of popliteal aneurysm with no visualization of a named outflow artery. The optimal management is
   A. Intravenous heparin
   B. Catheter-directed thrombolysis
   C. Emergency open repair
   D. Emergency stent graft repair

Correct Answer: B

3. The mortality of surgical repair for acute ischemia due to popliteal artery thrombosis is
   A. 1%
   B. 2%
   C. 3–3.5%
   D. Greater than 3.5%

Correct Answer: C

4. Most peripheral mycotic aneurysms in the lower extremity are caused by
   A. Bacterial endocarditis
   B. Intravenous drug abuse
   C. Open fracture of the tibia
   D. Infected below-knee PTFE grafts for arterial occlusive disease

Correct Answer: B

Chapter 15: Ruptured Popliteal Aneurysm

1. Rupture of popliteal aneurysm accounts for what percentage of patients operated on for PAA
   A. 5–7%
   B. 2–5%
   C. 2–3%
   D. Less than 2%

Correct Answer: B

2. The most common method of repair for a ruptured popliteal aneurysm is
   A. Endovascular repair
   B. Immediate open repair
   C. Hybrid repair
   D. Delayed open repair

Correct Answer: B

3. Endovascular repair for a rupture of proximal popliteal artery aneurysm is undertaken in an 89-year-old man with multiple comorbidities. He has two-vessel run-off. The following statement best reflects the outcome
   A. Endovascular repair should not have been undertaken.
   B. Hybrid repair with balloon occlusion of SFA via contralateral removal access followed by open repair.
   C. Immediate open repair.
   D. Endovascular repair using contralateral femoral access is superior in patients with two- to three-vessel runoff than in those with one-vessel run-off.

Correct Answer: D

4. The amputation rate following repair of a ruptured popliteal aneurysm is
   A. 9%
   B. 7%
   C. 5%
   D. Less than 5%

Correct Answer: A

Chapter 16: Infrapopliteal Artery Aneurysm

1. Infrapopliteal aneurysms are most associated with
   A. Sarcoidosis
   B. Ehlers-Danlos syndrome
   C. Marfan syndrome
   D. Intravenous drug abuse

Correct Answer: B

2. The most common complication of infrapopliteal artery aneurysm is
   A. Rupture
   B. Thrombosis and embolization
   C. Compression symptoms
   D. Development of arteriovenous fistula

Correct Answer: B

3. A 76-year-old man has 2.5 cm popliteal aneurysm and 1.0 cm tibioperoneal trunk aneurysm and has satisfactory GSV. The optimal management option is
   A. Surgical bypass for popliteal aneurysm and coil embolization for the tibioperoneal trunk aneurysm
   B. Surgical bypass for popliteal aneurysm and stent graft repair of the tibioperoneal trunk aneurysm
   C. Endovascular repair of popliteal and tibioperoneal trunk aneurysm
   D. Surgical bypass for popliteal artery aneurysm and tibioperoneal trunk aneurysm

Correct Answer: A

4. From Swedish vascular surgery, 235 legs with popliteal aneurysm presented with acute ischemia. Immediate surgery was performed in 135 legs including intraoperative thrombolysis in 32 cases. Thrombolysis was performed in 59 legs in the delayed surgery group. What was the amputation rate in each of these groups?
   A. 35% in the immediate surgery group and 14% in the delayed surgery group
   B. 30% in the immediate surgery group and 12% in the delayed surgery group
   C. 27% in the immediate surgery group and 7% in the delayed surgery group
   D. 20% in the immediate surgery group and 5% in the delayed surgery group

Correct Answer: C

5. The requirement for fasciotomy for (the two groups in question four) was
   A. 30% in the immediate surgery group and 11% in the delayed surgery group
   B. 25% in the immediate surgery group and 8% in the delayed surgery group
   C. 22% in the immediate surgery group and 6% in the delayed surgery group
   D. 20% in the immediate surgery group and 5% in the delayed surgery group

Correct Answer: A

Chapter 17: Popliteal Venous Aneurysm

1. The most plausible theory in the pathogenesis of popliteal venous aneurysm is
   A. Venous reflux and hypertension
   B. Inflammation
   C. Loss of focal normal connective tissue components in the vein wall
   D. Mechanical trauma

Correct Answer: C

2. The most helpful imaging study in planning the repair of popliteal venous aneurysm is
   A. Duplex venous ultrasound
   B. MRV
   C. CTV
   D. Venogram

Correct Answer: B

3. Complication rat following repair of popliteal venous aneurysm is
   A. 5%
   B. 10%
   C. 15%
   D. 20%

Correct Answer: D

4. Popliteal venous aneurysm should be repaired once the aneurysm reaches the diameter of
   A. 1.5 cm
   B. 2.0 cm
   C. 2.5 cm
   D. 3.0 cm

Correct Answer: B

Chapter 18: Management of Femoral Artery Pseudoaneurysm with AV Fistula

1. Acquired femoral arteriovenous fistula with a large communication result in
   A. Decrease in peripheral vascular resistance
   B. Increase in stroke volume
   C. Increase in heart rate
   D. Decrease in peripheral vascular resistance, increase in stroke volume, and increase in heart rate

Correct Answer: D

2. For the management of acquired femoral arteriovenous fistula, the imaging modality of choice is
   A. CTA
   B. MRA
   C. Catheter-based arteriography
   D. Color-duplex ultrasound

Correct Answer: C

3. Repair of acquired common femoral artery to common femoral vein fistula is best accomplished by
   A. Endovascular repair using stent graft
   B. Hybrid repair
   C. Open repair
   D. Endovascular repair using retractable coils

Correct Answer: C

4. Intraoperative successful repair of femoral arteriovenous fistula is confirmed by
   A. Arteriography
   B. Disappearance of thrill
   C. Intraoperative duplex imaging
   D. CTA in the hybrid operating room

Correct Answer: C

5. The common complication of open repair of acquired femoral artery-venous fistula is
   A. Excessive bleeding
   B. Surgical site infection
   C. Recurrence
   D. Excessive bleeding and surgical site infection

Common Answer: D

Chapter 19: Popliteal Artery and Venous Pseudoaneurysm with Arteriovenous Fistula

1. The common cause of AV fistula involving popliteal artery includes
   A. Congenital
   B. Knee arthroscopy
   C. Guidewire perforation during popliteal artery intervention for arterial occlusive disease
   D. Knee dislocation

Correct Answer: B

2. The imaging modality of choice for the management of popliteal artery venous fistula is
   A. Color-duplex ultrasound
   B. CTA
   C. MRA
   D. Catheter-based arteriography

Correct Answer: D

3. Popliteal arteriovenous fistula, at the joint line of recent onset, is a good risk; patient is best managed by
   A. Endovascular repair using covered stent
   B. Endovascular repair using detachable coils
   C. Open repair using posterior repair
   D. Open repair using medial approach

Correct Answer: C

Chapter 20: Lower Extremity Fasciotomy

1. The normal compartment pressure in the leg is
   A. 5–9 mmHg
   B. 10–12 mmHg
   C. 13–15 mmHg
   D. 16–18 mmHg

Correct Answer: B

2. For the diagnosis of compartment syndrome, the threshold used for compartment pressure is
   A. 19–20 mmHg
   B. 21–25 mmHg
   C. 25–29 mmHg
   D. 30 mmHg

Correct Answer: D

3. The strongest predictors for the need of fasciotomy in a patient with lower extremity trauma and arterial injury
   A. Ischemia time exceeding 6 h
   B. Ischemia time exceeding 2.5 h
   C. Rutherford category of arterial occlusion IIA or higher
   D. B and C

Correct Answer: D

4. The incidence of surgical site infection following fasciotomy is up to
   A. 25%
   B. 20%
   C. 15%
   D. 10%

Correct Answer: A

5. Early fasciotomy following acute vascular trauma results in
   A. Increased incidence of peroneal nerve palsy
   B. Increased incidence of surgical site infection
   C. Decreased incidence of surgical site infection
   D. Decreased incidence of secondary closure

Correct Answer: B

Chapter 21: Lower Extremity Major Amputations

1. Amputation proximal to the proximal third of the metatarsal shaft will result in which kind of deformity of the foot
   A. Permanent foot drop
   B. Equinus deformity
   C. Equinovarus deformity
   D. Skewfoot deformity

Correct Answer: B

2. In the absence of femoral pulse, the chance of healing of a below-the-knee amputation is
   A. Less than 10%
   B. Less than 15%
   C. Less than 20%
   D. Less than 25%

Correct Answer: D

3. Conversion rate of below-the-knee amputation to above-the-knee amputation is
   A. Less than 5%
   B. 5–10%
   C. 10–20%
   D. More than 20%

Correct Answer: C

4. The estimated mortality at 3 years following below-the-knee amputation for vascular disease is
   A. 20%
   B. 30%
   C. 37%
   D. Approximately, 43%

Correct Answer: D

5. The estimated energy expenditure for a patient with above-the-knee amputation is ________ as compared to 40% for below-the-knee amputation
   A. 70%
   B. 80%
   C. 85%
   D. 90%

Correct Answer: A

6. The perioperative mortality of above-the-knee amputation is
   A. 5–10%
   B. 11–18%
   C. 19–25%
   D. Greater than 25%

Correct Answer: B

7. The incidence of wound complication following hip disarticulation is
   A. 40%
   B. 50%
   C. 60%
   D. 70%

Correct Answer: C

Correction to: Contemporary Management of Lower Extremity Aneurysmal Disease

Correction to:
S. S. Hans, *Contemporary Management of Lower Extremity Aneurysmal Disease*,
https://doi.org/10.1007/978-3-032-00159-7

Owing to an unfortunate oversight, a preliminary version of the book was inadvertently published. The most important corrections are:

1. List of contributors holding affiliations for the commentary authors had been missed out and the same has been included.
2. The invited commentary content for Chapters 4 and 5 needs to be swapped. The text has been swapped and corrected in the revised publication.
3. The invited commentary author name along with their degrees under the header invited commentary for all chapters has been added.

The updated version of the book can be found at
https://doi.org/10.1007/978-3-032-00159-7

S. S. Hans, *Contemporary Management of Lower Extremity Aneurysmal Disease*,
https://doi.org/10.1007/978-3-032-00159-7_23

Index

S. S. Hans, *Contemporary Management of Lower Extremity Aneurysmal Disease*,
https://doi.org/10.1007/978-3-032-00159-7

C

D

E

F

MIX
Papier aus verantwortungsvollen Quellen
Paper from responsible sources
FSC® C105338

If you have any concerns about our products,
you can contact us on
ProductSafety@springernature.com

In case Publisher is established outside the EU,
the EU authorized representative is:
Springer Nature Customer Service Center GmbH
Europaplatz 3, 69115 Heidelberg, Germany

Printed by Libri Plureos GmbH
in Hamburg, Germany